BASIC HEALTH PUBLICATIONS USER'S GUIDE

TO INFLAMMATION, ARTHRITIS, AND AGING

Learn How Diet and Supplements Can Reduce Inflammation and Slow the Aging Process

D0908102

RONALD E. HUNNINGHAKE, M.D.

JACK CHALLEM Series Editor

The information contained in this book is based upon the research and personal and professional experiences of the author. It is not intended as a substitute for consulting with your physician or other healthcare provider. Any attempt to diagnose and treat an illness should be done under the direction of a healthcare professional.

The publisher does not advocate the use of any particular healthcare protocol but believes the information in this book should be available to the public. The publisher and author are not responsible for any adverse effects or consequences resulting from the use of the suggestions, preparations, or procedures discussed in this book. Should the reader have any questions concerning the appropriateness of any procedures or preparations mentioned, the author and the publisher strongly suggest consulting a professional healthcare advisor.

Series Editor: Jack Challem
Editor: Susan Andrews
Typesetter: Gary A. Rosenberg
Series Cover Designer: Mike Stromberg

Basic Health Publications User's Guides are published by Basic Health Publications, Inc.
28812 Top of the World Drive
Laguna Beach, CA 92651
949-715-7327

Copyright © 2005 Ronald E. Hunninghake, M.D.

ISBN: 1-59120-156-X

Printed in the United States of America

10   9   8   7   6   5   4   3   2   1

CONTENTS

INTRODUCTION

Are you in pain? Do you wake up stiff and tired each morning? Has your weight been creeping up in spite of your best efforts to control it? Is your doctor concerned about your cholesterol and blood pressure? Has a gnawing sense of depression been creeping into your life? Do you come from a family with arthritis or heart disease in its background?

If you find yourself answering "Yes" to many of these questions, there is hope. This health guide offers a new understanding that can help you overcome the symptoms of "bad" inflammation naturally. (A more complete list of questions is available in the "Bad" Inflammation Inventory at the end of Chapter 1.)

Most of us are familiar with acute inflammation: the redness and swelling that accompanies any painful injury or infection. We all get hurt from time to time. It's not unusual to get sick. We expect to heal.

But what if healing eludes us? What if pain persists or infection revisits us all too often? What if this protective system we once depended on now erodes our joints, plugs our arteries, and hurries our process of aging?

For the human species to survive, it had to have a competent inflammatory healing system. Otherwise injury and infection would have devastated our ancestors, given their primitive living conditions. Instead, experts have found the remains of early humans to be surprisingly free of disease. Something about the way they lived kept their inflammatory healing system sound.

Not so in modern America. Although we live longer than our ancestors, we do not live better. We are overweight, tired, and diabetic. Heart disease, rare in the nineteenth century, has now become our number-one killer. Our digestive systems are inflamed (acid blockers are the number-one selling drugs on the planet). Our joints hurt (more than 70 million Americans). We are fraught with allergies and asthma (56 million). Osteoporosis, macular degeneration, hepatitis, and hundreds of chronic "-itis" diseases plague us. We may be both the wealthiest and sickest society in history!

These chronic illnesses have a common denominator: inflammation! Not the healing kind mentioned earlier. This inflammation is "bad"! This is *chronic inflammation,* the kind that damages as it lingers. The "good" inflammation that helped our ancestors survive has turned "bad." This is why you hurt, why you are tired, and why you are at risk for silent diseases of aging.

This health guide will not only explore the *why* of this, but a very important *how:* how to heal your inflammatory system. You can overcome chronic inflammatory illness without resorting to costly anti-inflammatory medications with potentially life-threatening side effects.

You will learn what triggers "bad" inflammation, what regulates it, what balance factors you might be missing, and how dietary shifts have created it. Case studies will illustrate how implementing this new understanding can solve serious illness. You will rediscover our ancestral diet as well as five pathways to better health and slowed aging.

This health guide is based upon twenty-five years of caring for patients in a way that fostered their growth into *colearners*—that is, people who actively participate in their own healing. The colearner concept originated with the late Dr. Hugh Riordan, founder of the Center for the Improvement of Human Functioning International in Wichita, Kansas (also known as the Brightspot for Health, whose web address is www.brightspot.org). Practicing at this wonderful center under the direct tutelage of Dr. Riordan, I learned how to develop a caring, therapeutic relationship with my patients. As their preceptor, I asked them to become more involved in the detective work of discovering the underlying causes of their illnesses. Colearners assume responsibility for their health and well-being—and then go make it happen!

You can be a colearner too, and overcome the "bad" inflammation in your life. *Inflammation, Arthritis, and Aging* can serve as your guidebook.

CHAPTER 1

GOOD AND BAD INFLAMMATION

Remember the last time you cut yourself? Through a step-by-step process of recognition, response, and repair, your body proceeded to demonstrate its remarkable ability to heal.

Long ago ancient physicians studied this phenomenon of healing. They observed that the injury site appeared to get worse before it got better. Injuries became inflamed, then proceeded to heal.

As far back as the first century A.D., Celsus enumerated the four cardinal signs of inflammation: *swelling, redness, heat,* and *pain.* A century later, *loss of function* was added as the fifth key sign of inflammation.

These descriptive terms helped ancient physicians to *identify* inflammation. But it took the invention of the microscope to help modern physicians *understand* inflammation.

The Biology of Acute Inflammation

The five signs of inflammation are the visible manifestation of the body's highly orchestrated response to injury. Hidden from sight, five microscopic steps comprise the biology of *acute inflammation:*

- **Step 1—Trigger:** Bacteria that inhabit the skin or the object that broke the skin immediately invade the wound. Injury and the threat of infection *trigger* the inflammatory system.

- **Step 2—Activate:** Special messenger chemicals called cytokines are activated and released into the bloodstream.

- **Step 3—Mobilize:** The cytokines mobilize and

direct germ-fighting white blood cells to the injury site. The cytokines also loosen the junctions between the cells that comprise the blood vessel's wall.

Cytokine
A cell-communication molecule that regulates inflammatory activities.

- **Step 4—Eradicate:** The white cells migrate out into the arena of damaged tissue where the germs are methodically engulfed and eradicated through a process called *phagocytosis.* Damaged cellular debris is then cleaned up with powerful enzymes that are released from the white cells.

- **Step 5—Repair:** Finally, repair and growth chemicals from fibroblasts coordinate the replacement of damaged cells with scar tissue.

The word *acute* conveys a time frame that means "immediate." Acute care means care that is given right away. The body's inflammatory system treats the trigger threat as an immediate priority. Thanks to acute inflammation an infection is usually prevented, the wound is cleaned up, new cells are laid down, healthy scar formation occurs, and the body is returned to nearly 100 percent functionality.

Chronic Inflammation

But what about joint-destructive rheumatoid arthritis, those annoying seasonal allergies, the soaring rates of asthma, sports injuries that refuse to heal, decades-long dermatitis, unrelenting and sometimes bloody colitis, chronic sinusitis, and the insidious liver destruction of hepatitis C?

These are examples of conditions caused by *chronic inflammation.* Chronic is the opposite of acute. Acute gets right on the job—and gets it done! Chronic means that the job is prolonged and drawn out, often with adverse consequences. Healing is delayed and the imbalance responsible for the delay results in mounting injury.

In chronic inflammation, one or more inflammatory triggers will not go away. Either the irritant is entrenched like an environmental chemical exposure; or there is something repetitive involved, such as overuse injuries as occur in athletes or industrial workers; or perhaps a low-grade infection is smoldering somewhere in the body.

Such a chronic *trigger* puts the inflammatory system on perpetual *activation*. Excessive cytokines are generated day after day. More and more white cells are *mobilized* to the trigger site. An exaggerated effort to *eradicate* the unresolved trigger results in an ongoing release of an excess of tissue-damaging enzymes.

Surrounding tissues become innocently involved in free-radical damage that can trigger even more cytokine activation. In an ongoing effort to heal the inflamed area, *repair* chemicals accumulate in excess. Overexuberant scar formation clinically appears as granulation tissue, adhesions, or even keloids.

The five microscopic steps perversely malfunction in chronic inflammation. This pathologic predisposition to persistent inflammation is the basis of hundreds of diseases physicians identify with the "-itis" suffix. Arthritis is chronic joint inflammation. Colitis is chronic colon inflammation. Sinusitis is chronic inflammation of the sinuses, and so on. The list of chronic inflammatory illnesses has grown quite long in modern times.

Systemic Inflammation

Chronic inflammation does not lead to healing. The inflamed tissues remain inflamed, generally progressing into greater dysfunction and even destruction. The chronic inflammatory process, rather than staying localized to the area of injury, propagates throughout the body, triggering unhealthy changes in distant organs and tissues.

Jack Challem, in his groundbreaking book, *The Inflammation Syndrome*, describes this "radiating" effect as *systemic inflammation*. For example, the cardiovascular system (heart and blood vessels) is normally thought of as being distinct and separate from the gastrointestinal system (teeth, mouth, eso-

"Bad" Inflammation Inventory

1. Do you have seasonal allergies or a runny nose? — Y N
2. Do you get frequent colds or flu? — Y N
3. Do you have frequent skin problems or rashes? — Y N
4. Are you overweight by at least ten pounds? — Y N
5. Are you twenty pounds or more overweight? — Y N
6. Do you have achy stiff joints and/or muscles? — Y N
7. Do you use or have you used tobacco products? — Y N
8. Have you had a serious injury requiring a hospital stay? — Y N
9. Do you have bleeding or sore gums? — Y N
10. Do you sleep poorly? — Y N
11. Have you ever had a blood sugar reading over 100? — Y N
12. Do you have high blood pressure? — Y N
13. Do you eat ocean fish less than twice a week? — Y N
14. Do you live in a major metropolitan area? — Y N
15. Are you frequently stressed and depressed? — Y N
16. Do you exercise for less than twenty minutes three times per week? — Y N
17. Are you frequently exposed to pesticides? — Y N
18. Have you been diagnosed with any form of arthritis? — Y N
19. Are you asthmatic? — Y N
20. Do you have colitis, hepatitis, bronchitis, or any other "-itis"? — Y N

With each "yes" answer, you have an increased risk for low-grade, systemic inflammation.

phagous, stomach, intestines, and colon). Because of the radiating and spreading nature of chronic inflammation, malfunction of these unrelated organ systems can have cause and effect relationships that were previously unsuspected. It is now known that the inflammation of chronic gum infection (gingivitis) can trigger plaque formation in your arteries!

Systemic inflammation in its early stages is often referred to as *low-grade*, leaving it generally undetected. You may be aware that your gums get sore from time to time and bleed. You won't be aware of the involvement of the walls of your arteries. The chronic infection can trigger a buildup of arterial plaque, silently putting you at greater risk for a sudden heart attack or stroke.

Low-grade inflammation can smolder for years in your brain, silently setting the stage for Alzheimer's. It can cause subtle but progressive changes in your retina, one day manifesting as decreased central vision (macular degeneration). A growing body of research now suggests that low-grade, systemic inflammation plays a major role in *all* degenerative illness.

The key unanswered question here is: Why does acute inflammation become chronic and systemic? Why does a bodily mechanism that was meant to repair injury and protect us from infection, perpetuate and spread injury instead? What makes "good" inflammation turn "bad"?

Inflammation is of itself neither good nor bad. Without inflammation we could not survive. In this sense, inflammation is definitely good. When the inflammatory mechanism goes out of balance and turns chronic or systemic then it is bad for our health.

CHAPTER 2

INFLAMMATORY TRIGGERS

Remember that cut we were talking about? That acted as a trigger to the inflammatory process. The injury to your skin and the pain it produced immediately *activated* the release of the chemical messengers called *cytokines*. The bacteria that flooded in to contaminate the wound also acted as an inflammatory trigger. By definition, a trigger sets off or activates a process or mechanism.

The many triggers that activate inflammation can be categorized into several recognizable groups:

- **Physical injuries:**

  Acute: cuts, lacerations, burns, broken bones, hypoxemia

  Chronic: athletic injuries, traumatic and overuse injuries

- **Infections:**

  Acute: colds, flu, pneumonia, pink eye, wound infection

  Chronic: sinusitis, parasitic, toenail fungus, Hepatitis C virus

- **Environmental toxins and irritants:**

  Acute: thick dust, toxic inhalants, cold air, exercise, irritants

  Chronic: chemicals, air pollution, cigarette smoke, chemicals released from new carpets (carpet out-gassing), lung irritants

- **Allergies and sensitivities:**

  Acute: foods (hives, anaphylactic shock)

  Chronic: foods (sensitivities that involve multiple

systems), dusts, molds, pollens, grasses, trees, animal danders, dust mites, cigarette smoke, perfumes, salicylates, sulfites, others

Acute vs. Chronic Triggers

Acute triggers are immediate and short-lived. They serve as appropriate activators of the inflammatory response, and then their job is over. The activation signal fades. The step-by-step microscopic response unfolds in its proper sequence and the job of healing is accomplished.

Chronic triggers also activate the inflammatory cascade; only here the job is inappropriately prolonged. As with an acute trigger, the cytokine signal to activate the inflammatory response is sent out. But with a chronic trigger, that signal is sent over and over again.

The inflammatory response does not differentiate between the true threat of an acute trigger, and the repeating false alarm of a chronic trigger. Chronic triggers can range from harmless irritants to smoldering low-grade infections that repeatedly activate inflammation and never shut off. The result is chronic inflammation with subsequent damage to the involved tissues.

A Case of Allergies

About two years prior to writing this guide, I began experiencing the following symptoms. My nose would start to run and my head felt a bit congested. I waved off the symptoms as "a touch of hay fever." As time went on, things got worse. Every few weeks, the dam broke and my nose drained profusely. Those were the two-box tissue days.

As a wellness-oriented doctor who saw many patients, it was embarrassing and distracting. I joked about it, but actually felt very helpless. The symptoms would usually crescendo into a full-blown upper respiratory infection. I would get better, only to have the cycle repeat itself a few weeks later. One patient commented frankly: "Doctor, you need to see a doctor!"

Why had I developed nasal allergies? In the past, an occasional glass of red wine would make me sneeze; otherwise I had been immune to environmental triggers. I had continued to work in the same office. I had lived in the same house for more than twelve years. What was triggering my nasal allergies?

The allergy symptoms were debilitating enough to require strong antihistamine medication. This proved insufficient. I added a potent intranasal steroid to cool my inflamed nasal lining. Medication and large doses of oral vitamin C finally helped me to subdue the symptoms, but not eliminate them. I awoke each morning to a stopped-up nose. Fifteen to twenty minutes of exasperating nose blowing would allow me to breathe a little better—for a little while.

Unable to identify a causative trigger and faced with a poor response to medication, I found myself backed into a therapeutic corner.

Allergic Rhinitis

More than 40 million allergic rhinitis sufferers fight this annoying disease daily. Stuffed up nose, itchy eyes, poor sleep, dark circles under the eyes, irritability, and the frequent progression to ear, sinus, throat, and lung infections are symptoms of rhinitis. The cause of this malady is typically laid at the feet of *chronic environmental triggers*. It is a medical truism that *chronic triggers cause chronic inflammation*. Because the chronic environmental triggers are difficult to avoid, pharmacologic treatment begins with an attempt to block the alert-signal that these triggers activate, namely *cytokines*.

Allergic Rhinitis

An inflammatory condition of the nasal passages triggered by environmental allergens and characterized by swelling, irritation, and drainage from the nose.

Histamine is the main activating cytokine for the symptoms of allergic rhinitis. Antihistamines block this activation. Side effects of antihistamines (such as Benadryl) include excessive drying of mucous membranes and drowsiness. Improved antihistamines (such as Allegra) are less likely to cause drowsiness but are expensive. Cromolyn sodium is a mast cell stabilizing drug that prevents histamines from being released.

Leukotriene blockers (such as Singulair) go beyond histamine blockers. From the emerging science of cell membrane function, we now know that leukotrienes activate inflammation. The precursors for leukotrienes are derived from long-chain fatty acids found in the diet. Fatty acids are converted into leukotrienes by an enzyme located in the cell membrane called *5-lipoxygenase* (LOX). Furthermore, leukotrienes are part of a family of cellular regulators known as *eicosanoids*. Their role in inflammation is enormously important.

Eicosanoids
A class of compounds (such as prostaglandins), derived from polyunsaturated fatty acids found in the diet. Eicosanoids are synthesized in cell membranes and have important cell-regulating functions.

Eicosanoids are synthesized in the cell membrane and released; they do their job and self-destruct in mere seconds. Cytokines activate inflammation. Eicosanoids regulate inflammation. Cytokine and eicosanoid-blocker medications modulate and control inflammation. Rarely do they totally solve the problem of chronic triggers and runaway chronic inflammation.

Steroids are considered the ultimate inflammation modulator because they block all cytokines and all eicosanoids. This means that high-dose steroids can shut down both bad and good inflammation. Shutting down bad inflammation can aid in the treatment of many "-itis" diseases. Unfortunately, the protective effect of good inflammation is lost and serious side effects can ensue. The goal is to use the least amount of steroid that will control the specific "bad" inflammation. Intranasal steroid sprays accomplish this by limiting exposure to the surface membranes inside the nose. Systemic side effects rarely occur.

At the height of my own allergic rhinitis, my desperate attempts to control the overwhelming symptoms had escalated to using four medications:

Nasalcrom, a mast cell stabilizer; Allegra, an antihistamine; Singulair, a leukotriene-blocker; and Flonase, a nasal steroid. My symptoms diminished but would not disappear.

I thought I might be getting a handle on things when one day the pain in my sinuses showed up. Then when I blew my nose, there were streaks of blood and yellow mucus. My allergies were progressing to a sinus infection!

Arthritis

Allergic rhinitis has known inflammatory triggers. In many chronic inflammatory conditions the initiating triggers are not as obvious, as in the case of arthritis.

Seventy million Americans have painful, inflamed joints. Osteoarthritis is the most prevalent form. What triggers osteoarthritis? It begins with wear and tear of the joint cartilage pad. The cartilage wears away until there is nothing to cushion and lubricate the movements of the articulating bones. Silent and progressive trauma damages the connecting surfaces of the bones, triggering the release of inflammation-activating cytokines. White blood cells are mobilized, move in, and accumulate. They produce an overabundance of tissue-destructive enzymes that form free radicals. Free radicals cause slow erosion of the joint tissues. Over time, the classic symptoms of inflammation make their appearance in the form of pain, swelling, disability, bone spurs, and joint deformities.

Other forms of arthritis, like rheumatoid arthritis (RA), are more dramatic and severely damaging. The immune system forms antibodies that cross-react with the synovial capsule of certain joints. This results in an aggressive response of the white blood cells. Severe and painful deformities of the afflicted joints ensue, sometimes requiring joint replacement surgery. In an effort to quell the rampant destruction of RA, powerful immune-suppressant medications such as methotrexate are utilized. Methotrexate is also used as a chemotherapeutic agent against cancer.

Steroidals and Nonsteroidals

More than 250 drugs have been used to treat the various forms of arthritis. The most commonly prescribed are the *nonsteroidal anti-inflammatory drugs* (NSAIDs). These are the doctor's anti-inflammatory workhorses. They are mildly effective, though their safety has come into question in recent years.

NSAIDs were designed to control inflammation without the side effects of high-dose steroids. Sadly, while less prone to side effects than steroids, NSAIDs have their own list of concerns. Ironically, though given to treat inflammation, they can end up *inflaming* the lining of the stomach and intestine. Gastritis, ulcers, and intestinal inflammation can occur in 50 percent of users. This can lead to pain, bleeding, and increased permeability of the intestinal membranes (sometimes referred to as *leaky gut*). Heart failure, heart attack, stroke, kidney disease, and other blood platelet disorders can develop as serious side effects of this class of meds.

Steroids are a class of compounds that are naturally made by the adrenal gland. Hydrocortisone is an adrenal steroid. Steroids (such as prednisone) are also made synthetically in the laboratory and are available as medication. The pharmaceutical use of synthetic steroids mimics the adrenal gland's response to stress. This imitation is up to twenty times more powerful than nature's maximum effect and is fraught with dangerous side effects if used chronically.

Hydrocortisone is the adrenal's stress adaptation steroid. Approximately 30–40 milligrams of hydrocortisone is made by the adrenal glands each day to help us cope with life-stress. That amount can double during serious stress, such as illness or grave injury. In fact, increased hydrocortisone production is a natural component of the body's inflammatory response. Hydrocortisone is anti-inflammatory, yet the body utilizes it as a self-preserving countermeasure to balance and modulate the destructive forces that are invoked during an inflammatory response. This illustrates the importance of balance in the inflammatory equation.

Cyclooxygenase—COX

Aspirin, ibuprofen, and other NSAIDs work by inhibiting the activity of the cellular enzyme *cyclooxygenase* (COX). Thanks to extensive research by pharmaceutical companies, much is known about COX. There are two forms of cyclooxygenase: COX-1 and COX-2. COX-1 was found to be an important regulator of an array of biological functions including blood pressure, body temperature, stomach integrity, circulation, clotting, and many more essential functions, including inflammation. Researchers believe that the body maintains steady levels of COX-1 to attend to these functions.

In the 1990s, COX-2 was discovered as an inflammation-specific enzyme. Celebrex and Vioxx were developed to specifically inhibit the COX-2 enzyme. They were marketed as *selective COX-2 inhibitors*. Theoretically, COX-2 inhibitors would have fewer gastrointestinal side effects compared to the traditional COX-1-inhibiting NSAIDs.

Unfortunately, COX-2 inhibitors turned out to be only 20 percent selective. Twenty percent of their function was limited to COX-2 inflammation. That meant that 80 percent of their anti-inflammatory effect was similar to the old COX-1 NSAIDs, and that included similar side effects.

A more sinister problem emerged regarding the COX-2 inhibitors. One study comparing Vioxx to the older COX-1 NSAID, naproxen, found a four times greater incidence of heart attacks. This and more recent studies prompted the maker of Vioxx to remove it from the market in 2004. The side effects of other NSAIDs have since come under suspicion, also.

Understanding Inflammation

When the COX enzymes are inhibited with NSAIDs, there is a relatively high incidence of side effects. Side effects are the price we pay when we choose medicines that block fundamental biochemical pathways in our desperate attempt to relieve symptoms. Multiple side effects imply *interference* with fundamental biochemical functions.

Inflammation is one of many important biologic functions. Given the destructive power of inflammation, proper balance between pro-inflammatory activators and anti-inflammatory regulators must be maintained for surrounding cells to survive. COX enzymes produce both anti- and pro-inflammatory eicosanoids that balance and modulate the inflammatory process.

Controlling inflammatory triggers with medication had not given me adequate relief from my chronic inflammatory rhinitis. I could not figure out why I was reacting to mystery triggers while others in the same environment were not. Something was predisposing me to rhinitis. Something was causing my cells to produce more pro-inflammatory eicosanoids than anti-inflammatory ones. That something was throwing my system out of balance and predisposing me to the "bad" inflammation of chronic rhinitis.

I happened to review some personal lab work I had done a few years prior to the onset of my illness. I discovered two results that put me on the right path to solving this mystery.

CHAPTER 3

BIOLOGIC REGULATORS

I had tried to solve my escalating allergy symptoms with pharmacologic thinking. It wasn't working. So my attention turned to biologic thinking. I was overresponding to inflammatory triggers common in the home and at work. Many other people in my family and at work were not overresponding to these same triggers. What made my inflammatory response different?

Understanding C-Reactive Protein

My allergic symptoms began sometime in 2001. I can't remember exactly when they began, because the onset was so gradual. It began with a slightly runny nose with occasional flare-ups that acted like a one-day cold. I had not yet entered the troubling phase of my illness. Not surprisingly, I overlooked the importance of a little known test I had done on myself: the *C-reactive protein* (CRP).

CRP is a byproduct of a specific cytokine called *interleukin-6* (IL-6). IL-6 is a potent inflammatory activator. Liver and abdominal fat cells process IL-6 into CRP. At first researchers believed that CRP was an inert metabolic byproduct with no ability to activate inflammation. Current research suggests that CRP is a full-fledged inflammation-activating cytokine.

The CRP test had been around since the 1930s. Rheumatologists used it to help diagnose rheumatoid arthritis and other highly in-

C-Reactive Protein (CRP) Test
A protein test that measures the level of inflammation going on in the body. The test is nonspecific: it does not indicate where the inflammation is coming from.

flammatory autoimmune disorders. The low sensitivity of the original CRP was only adequate to measure *acute* or *high-grade chronic* inflammation or serious infection. Recently a more sensitive CRP test became available that could detect *low-grade, systemic* inflammation.

The highly sensitive CRP could pick up what was previously undetected by the old CRP: hidden inflammation. For the first time doctors began to realize that systemic inflammation was a major underlying factor in chronic degenerative illness. (See Table 3.1.) The biggest surprise came in the field of cardiology.

TABLE 3.1. COMMON HEALTH CONDITIONS ASSOCIATED WITH ELEVATED CRP LEVELS

Conditions	CRP levels
Abdominal fat	Produces CRP; fat is pro-inflammatory
Alzheimer's disease	Elevates CRP and homocysteine
Asthma	Inflammation in airways raises CRP
Cancers	Can elevate CRP; not diagnostic
Diabetes (types 1 & 2)	Elevates CRP; associated with obesity
Fibromyalgia	CRP often elevated
Gingivitis	Elevates CRP; a risk factor for heart disease
Lupus	Classic CRP elevation in this auto-immune disease
Metabolic Syndrome X	Elevates CRP; epidemic in America
Psoriasis	Elevated CRP; cytokines come from skin
Rheumatoid arthritis	Marked elevation (can exceed 100)
Severe trauma	Marked elevation (can exceed 100)
Smoking addiction	Raises CRP
Stroke	CRP correlates with higher blood viscosity

The CRP Predicts Heart Attack

In the early 1990s, Dr. B.C. Berk and colleagues first described CRP elevation in patients with *unstable angina*. Cardiologists define unstable angina as a changing chest pain pattern indicative of impending heart attack. At that time, heart and blood vessel disease was not considered inflammatory in nature. Doctor Berk's study suggested that angina had an inflammatory component. In 1994, Dr. G. Liuzzo showed that an elevated CRP in unstable angina reliably predicted long-term outcome: the higher the CRP, the worse the prognosis.

Later studies showed that an elevated CRP could predict a heart attack *six to eight years in advance*! To cap it off, Dr. Paul Ridker compared the predictive value of CRP to the gold standard of heart disease prediction: the LDL "bad" cholesterol. Dr. Ridker showed that a high CRP was a better predictor of heart disease than a high LDL. Some cardiologists are now referring to CRP as the "golden marker" for high-risk inflammatory changes in coronary arteries.

These exciting findings led the center where I practice medicine to offer the CRP to our employees in 2001 to help us better assess our risk for heart disease using this new tool. My CRP was moderately elevated at 1.7 milligrams (mg) per liter. Table 3.2 describes the risk stratification of the CRP as it relates to future heart attack.

TABLE 3.2. CRP "RISK" FOR HEART DISEASE	
CRP Levels	**Risk**
< 0.7	Lowest Risk
0.7 – 1.1	Low Risk
1.2 – 1.9	Moderate Risk
2.0 – 3.8	High Risk
> 3.8	Highest Risk

If the CRP were specific for coronary inflammation, this result would have suggested that I was at moderate risk for hidden heart disease. However, the

CRP is a *nonspecific* biologic marker for low-grade, systemic inflammation. Elevated levels point to hidden inflammation—unfortunately the CRP cannot tell you where the inflammation is coming from!

In my case, the inflammation was not hidden. My moderately elevated CRP indicated allergies, not hidden artery disease. Other than being a male, I had zero-risk factors for heart disease: negative family and smoking history, low blood pressure, normal weight, and low lipids; I was fairly fit, and had normal exercise stress tests and a near-normal calcium score using electron beam tomography to assess my coronary arteries in 2002.

Was this elevated CRP the clue I was looking for? Cytokines are biologic regulators. CRP is a cytokine. Did my elevated CRP suggest an imbalance of cytokines? It made me question whether "bad" inflammation was itself an imbalance of cytokines.

Following the Cytokine Cascade

Inflammation is only one of many important biologic functions that are regulated by cytokines. Cytokines bind to specific membrane receptors to signal the cell to change its behavior via gene expression.

Cytokine is a general name for a whole family of "-kines." Triggers activate the cytokines "to act on cells." *Chemokines* act by mobilizing and attracting white blood cells to the area of injury. *Lymphokines* are made by lymphocytes to direct the immune response. *Interleukin* is another cytokine regulator; made by one white cell, it acts on another to coordinate phagocytosis and foreign protein eradication. Cytokines direct fibroblasts in the repair process. All five of the microscopic steps of inflammation are influenced and regulated by cytokines.

Cytokines may act on the cells that secrete them (*autocrine*); or on nearby cells (*paracrine*); or even on distant cells (*endocrine*). Cytokines often are produced and act in a cascade in which target cells are activated to make sequential cytokines. Cytokines are made by many cell types, most commonly the helper T cells and macrophages (two important types of immune cells). Helper T cells are important in localized inflammatory responses.

Although *synergistic cytokines* can cascade and act together to produce a specific action like activation of inflammation, *antagonistic cytokines* counterbalance the inflammatory response. Antagonistic cytokines compete for the same receptors as synergistic cytokines or use other mechanisms to produce an antagonizing action. Antagonistic cytokines help to regulate inflammation and keep it from spiraling totally out of control.

Wait a minute! "Out of control!" That sounded like my allergies! Did I lack antagonistic cytokines? Did my nasal mucosal lining exist in a *net* pro-inflammatory cytokine environment? Was this predisposing me to this excessive inflammation?

Sentinels Out of Balance

In its role as sentinel, the inflammatory system is constantly poised to go into action. Any bodily tissue can generate pro-inflammatory cytokines at the slightest provocation. To hold this readiness state in check, there must be a counterbalance control system in the body. Anti-inflammatory mechanisms must exist to regulate pro-inflammatory forces.

My elevated CRP was one clue in a complicated scavenger hunt. Something was triggering my pro-inflammatory cytokine alarm system inappropriately. The elevated CRP pointed me in the direction of an inflammatory system out of balance and out of control. Pro-inflammatory cytokines were exceeding anti-inflammatory cytokines. I began to visualize "bad" inflammation as an excess of pro-inflammatory cytokines. Pro-inflammatory excess is at the root of chronic and systemic inflammatory illnesses.

The Grassfire Analogy

Inflammation can be compared to a grassfire. Imagine a field of grass that is dried out due to excessive sunshine (pro-inflammatory cytokines). A match is thrown onto the field of dried-out grass (inflammatory trigger). One small match is enough to trigger a very destructive grassfire (acute inflammation) that can then burn down and continue to smolder (chronic inflammation).

Now, if the field has had adequate rainfall (anti-inflammatory cytokines) the grass will be generally green and healthy. That same match (inflammatory trigger) will do nothing other than light small areas of dryness. The match (a trigger) is not the cause of a big fire. *The fire of inflammation is triggered only if a predisposition already exists.*

The balance between sunshine and rainfall regulates this predisposition. Sunshine is a profire regulator and rainfall is an antifire regulator. In this sense, pro-inflammatory cytokines like sunshine are not "bad!" The field needs sunshine, just as our bodies need the protection of acute pro-inflammatory cytokines. It is only when a *chronic imbalance* between pro- and anti-inflammatory cytokines *predisposes* the body to chronic and systemic inflammation that you and I are at risk for an "-itis" illness.

This analogy made it clear that "bad" inflammation is caused by an imbalance of cytokines. An excess of pro-inflammatory cytokines such as CRP and IL-6 tips the scales toward damaging inflammation. But why does this excess develop? Is there a *balance factor* that regulates this tendency? Cytokines regulate inflammation, but what regulates the cytokines?

My essential fatty acid test results gave me my next major clue in this mystery.

CHAPTER 4

BALANCE FACTORS

The second fortuitous test that I had run in July of 2001 was an essential fatty acid panel. This is a blood test of the omega-3, omega-6, and omega-9 fats in the test subject's red blood cell membranes. The omega fats are what nutritionists call "*good fats.*" They are essential: the body cannot synthesize them; they must be obtained in the diet. Many mis-informed experts mistakenly consider *all fats* to be "bad." There are good fats and there are bad fats. There are also fats that exist in the gray zone between "good" and "bad."

Good Fats/Bad Fats

Omega-9 oils are found in nuts and olives, both of which are getting good press with all the positive research on the Mediterranean diet. Omega-6 oils are found in seeds and grains. Omega-6 oils are used extensively in processed and packaged foods. Although omega-6s are essential in nature, the nutri-tional reviews on these oils are coming in mixed.

Manufacturers have learned how to purposely pressurize and heat omega-6 oils to give them a longer shelf life. This hydrogenation process in which liquid oils are solidified or are partially solidified cre-ates *trans fats*, the current villain in nutritional circles. Saturated fats are also solid at room temperature and are found primarily in animal-based foods. A substan-tial body of research would put saturated fats in the "bad fats" circle. Others believe that the disease-causing potential of saturated fats depends on the quality of foods consumed with these fats. Meat, which is high in saturated fat, may become a "bad" fat when it is consumed in the presence of large amounts of refined carbohydrates such as sugar and white flour. Lowering one's saturated fat intake too much has been associated with a higher incidence of stroke.

The uncontested hero of this melodrama is omega-3, best obtained from ocean seafood, and to a limited extent from flax and various nuts. Omega-3 fats, along with omega-6, are nutrient precursors to an important group of short-lived hormones called eicosanoids. Eicosanoids are synthesized from omega-3 and omega-6 in all cell membranes. The eicosanoids perform the crucial task of regulating cytokines. Modern research has demonstrated numerous health benefits from consuming adequate omega-3.

Was omega-3 "the balance factor" I was looking for that regulated cytokines and inflammatory health?

"Within Normal Limits"

Since 1993, I had regularly used our center's lab to assess my essential fatty acid levels. With the exception of a low omega-6 fat called *gamma linolenic acid* (GLA), I believed my levels were "within normal limits" during this time span. I can now see that I was mistaken.

The reference levels that establish what is a "normal value" for any given lab test are established from a population of patients who are having their blood tested at that lab. My fatty acid levels were "normal" in reference to the *standard deviation curve* of the typical Americans we were seeing at our center. Typical Americans were eating a typical American diet. "Normal" was being defined by the modern dietary cuisine. I was wrong to assume that the modern diet delivers anywhere near optimal fatty acid levels.

Standard Deviation Curve
Standard deviation is the statistical distribution of a population along a mathematical curve used to assess what is normal or not normal for that population.

In particular, I am referring to two specific readings on my test results: the *arachidonic acid* (AA) and *eicosapentaenoic acid* (EPA) levels. The ratio of these two omega fats regulates eicosanoid function at the cellular level. An excess of AA in the diet, or a deficiency of EPA intake creates an unfavorable ratio that promotes excessive inflammation.

AA Is Pro-inflammatory

AA is produced from the omega-6 precursor: *linoleic acid*. Linoleic acid is essential for health, and is found in vegetable oils such as corn, safflower, peanut, and soy, and in packaged foods containing these oils. Unfortunately, the consumption of excess linoleic acid leads to the excess production of AA. AA is then converted into a powerful pro-inflammatory eicosanoid called *prostaglandin E_2*.

The eicosanoids are very powerful but short-lived hormonal regulators in the body. ("Eicos" is Greek for "twenty.") Eicosanoids are twenty-carbon molecules. There are hundreds of eicosanoids that function in the vicinity of cell membranes. Picture the cell as a beehive. The eicosanoids are like the bees flying out into the near vicinity of the hive to gather information for the good of the hive. The eicosanoids perform many important functions that promote cellular health. Blood pressure, clotting, mucus production, body temperature, circulation, and immunity are a few of the bodily processes that eicosanoids regulate.

Eicosanoids are the cytokine regulators that keep "good" and "bad" inflammation in balance. Our dietary intake of fatty acids regulates the production of eicosanoids. An excess of omega-6 fats in the diet creates a pro-inflammatory imbalance. This imbalance affects every cell in the body!

More EPA Is Anti-inflammatory

AA is converted into pro-inflammatory prostaglandin E_2 by our old friend cyclooxygenase (COX). COX also converts EPA into prostaglandins E_1 and E_3, which are anti-inflammatory. COX is the rate-limiting step. EPA competes with AA for the COX enzyme.

If there is an excess of AA in the diet, the available

COX enzyme molecules will be occupied primarily with the AA molecule. AA tends to be converted to pro-inflammatory eicosanoids rapidly. The structure of the AA molecule makes it a good "fit" in the COX enzyme and the chemical transformation occurs quickly.

EPA molecules are similar to AA molecules with one exception: EPA fits differently into the COX enzyme. COX can still transform EPA into eicosanoids, but the process is *slower*. More EPA molecules occupying more COX enzymes slow down the formation of pro-inflammatory eicosanoids. This effectively makes EPA "anti-inflammatory."

If your diet contains an excess of AA molecules, COX dishes you out an excess of pro-inflammatory prostaglandins. By increasing your dietary or supplemental intake of EPA molecules, your COX enzymes get tied up and slowed down. Fewer pro-inflammatory prostaglandins are made, and more of the anti-inflammatory species result. AA/EPA is the crucial cytokine-balancing ratio!

My Breakthrough!

My own AA/EPA ratio in July of 2001 was 17/1. As the inflammatory rhinitis progressively worsened, I happened to recheck that number in March of 2002. It was still 17/1. Frustrated, I kept looking for a way to reduce this escalating inflammatory process.

About this time our center began carrying pharmaceutical-grade fish oil capsules. Years before I had tried to take our standard brand unsuccessfully. I could never get past "the fish burp." Rancid fish oils don't digest well. Some people have the stomach to do it. I didn't. Even freezing the capsules in advance didn't work. I knew from research that I *should* take them. But my stomach didn't care about the research.

The molecularly distilled, mercury-free and PCB-free, pharmaceutical-grade fish oil was a breath of fresh air. No burp. No aftertaste. I could get down four to six capsules a day without difficulty. To my delight and great relief, the allergies began to recede.

In April of 2004 I had my next AA/EPA ratio done: 5/1! A follow-up CRP done at that same time was now down to 0.6 milligrams per liter. Best of all, my morning ritual of nose blowing was a thing of the past. I could breathe and sleep freely again without the need for medication.

Other Balance Factors

At first I thought that increasing my fish oil intake was the only reason I had gotten better. Careful reflection reminded me of several other contributing factors that I need to mention.

One of the many tests offered by the laboratory at the center is the cytotoxic test. This is a fasting blood test where the fresh specimen is spun down and the white cells are separated. Small amounts of ninety common foods or food antigens are dried and placed in the wells of test slides. The patient's white cells are added to each of these slides and allowed to incubate for three hours. Each slide is microscopically read and scored according to the degree of cytotoxicity on a scale of 0 to 4. The "0" means there is no reaction of your white cells to that food. The numbers from "1" all the way up to "4" indicate that your white cells react adversely to the food with a "1" being a mild reaction, "2" and "3" being moderate reactions, and "4" being a severe reaction. Conventional immunologists and allergists have ridiculed the cytotoxic test for decades. However, our lab has provided clinically consistent and reliable results for more than twenty-five years. A well-trained, certified medical technician is a prerequisite for results that can be trusted. The results are given to each of our patient-colearners in an appointment setting where they can be interpreted in the context of the patient's illness and overall clinical picture.

My Cytotoxic Results

Around the time I started taking extra fish oil, I had a cytotoxic retest done. Years earlier I had tested "0" and nonreactive to wheat. This was in spite of a positive family history for celiac disease. Celiac disease results from a severe reaction to the gluten in wheat. In the full-blown version of celiac disease, the patient suffers diarrhea and malabsorption. It is estimated that there are many more sufferers of partial gluten sensitivity where the resulting symptoms are less specific.

My more recent cytotoxic test registered "2" for wheat. Something had changed. I wondered if this could be a partial explanation for my development of nasal allergies? So I went off wheat products. Soon I noticed I was less bloated and gassy. My digestion seemed better. The nasal symptoms began to diminish.

Another change that deserves mention was the addition of quercetin to my supplement program. Quercetin is a bioflavonoid derivative of apples and onions. It is known for its potent anti-inflammatory effect. It is especially good for allergies of both airway and gastrointestinal origins. It is a powerful antioxidant.

My records show I first started taking quercetin with bromelain (to enhance absorption of the quercetin and because bromelain has anti-inflammatory properties of its own) about four months prior to the cessation of my severe allergy symptoms.

Also at this time I began teaching a series of weekly lectures and a weekly seminar on the Atkins' Diet. To teach something effectively, one must try to live it as well. This meant eliminating the remaining elements of refined sugar, refined grains, and unhealthy fats that lurked in various snack foods. Over a two- to three-month period I lost about twelve pounds that had insidiously found their way around my waist. I was able to comfortably tighten my belt by an extra two notches.

Summary of Changes

My severe allergic rhinitis, which had been so unresponsive to four major medications, *completely ceased* with the adoption of the following changes:

- an increased intake of pharmaceutical-grade fish oil

- a resulting improvement of my AA/EPA ratio, from 17:1 to 5:1

- the elimination of wheat from my diet

- the addition of quercetin with bromelain as a supplement

- the elimination of sugar, refined grains, and separated oils

- the subsequent reduction in my CRP from 1.7 to 0.6 milligrams per liter.

This left me with another big question: Had I improved due to one significant change or was it due to the synergistic effect of all these changes taken together? The holistic approach to health care has a major weakness from the scientific perspective: too many variables happening all at once! It seemed too complicated to sort out until I began to look at things from a larger perspective.

A big share of why I had gotten better had come from my dietary changes. It would only make sense that something as pervasive and fundamental as diet might explain why chronic inflammatory disease was on the rise in the general population. I started to look at how the modern diet had changed over the last several thousand years!

CHAPTER 5

PRO-INFLAMMATORY DIETARY SHIFTS

I thought about the changes I had made in my diet. It reminded me of a lecture I had given on the demise of our ancestral diet and how it related to the rise in inflammation in modern times. Our ancestral diet is not really a diet *per se*; rather it is a description of how our ancient ancestors used to eat. It stretches back before the advent of agriculture, several thousands of years ago.

In my lecture I defined the nutritional structure of the ancestral diet with four measurable characteristics:

- **Wholeness**—foods eaten as they once grew, without significant change to their cellular content.

- **Omega-6/Omega-3**—the ratio of omega-6 fats to omega-3 fats consumed, with a 1:1 ratio being the norm for that period.

- **Glycemic Index**—a measure of a food's tendency to stimulate the release of insulin.

- **ORAC Score**—a measurement of the free-radical scavengering power of a food; its antioxidant strength.

The ancestral diet itself was 100 percent whole, with an ideal omega-6/omega-3 ratio of 1:1; it had a very low glycemic index, and a high ORAC score. How do we know that these are the characteristics of the way our ancestors ate? We know them thanks to the outstanding work of Dr. S. Boyd Eaton.

Our Ancestral Diet

In 1985, S. Boyd Eaton, M.D., of Emory University,

Atlanta, published a watershed article in the *New England Journal of Medicine*. This article summarized a vast body of anthropologic and archaeological evidence that had been derived from the ethnographic records of 229 "hunter-gatherer" cultures. In particular, Dr. Eaton characterized the diet of our primitive ancestors.

Our ancestors were hunters of animal foods and gatherers of plant foods. Eaton showed that 73 percent of the studied societies obtained *more than half* of their food from hunting animals and fish. Their remaining caloric needs were met with gathering a large variety of plant matter, including leaves, roots, fruits, berries, seeds, and nuts. Paleopathologic techniques were used to assess fossil remains. The stunning conclusion? Primitive hunter-gatherers generally were healthier than people are now and they rarely experienced degenerative/inflammatory disease.

Given the rampant obesity, inflammation, and degenerative disease found in modern Western culture today, we are faced with three compelling questions: How has the human diet changed over the course of history? Have these changes been beneficial? If not, what can we do to modify our food choices to recapture the benefits of our "ancestral diet"?

Four Dietary Epochs

Four great historical shifts in the human diet tell the story of the rise of chronic inflammation. Four human epochs comprise this history of diet:

1. Hunter-gatherer

2. Agricultural

3. Industrial

4. Fast Food

As the human diet has changed in each epoch so has the increased tendency for pro-inflammatory illness to occur. Table 5.1 defines the rather profound changes in the human diet that have occurred with each passing epoch.

TABLE 5.1. PRO-INFLAMMATORY DIETARY SHIFTS				
Dietary Epoch	**Whole-ness**	**Omega-6:3**	**Glycemic**	**ORAC**
Hunter-gatherer	100%	1:1	Very low	High
Agricultural	90%	5:1	Low	Medium
Industrial	60%	10:1	Medium	Low
Fast Food	40%	20:1	High	Very low

In Chapter 4, Balance Factors, it became apparent that the omega-6/omega-3 ratio has a profound impact on "bad" inflammation. Could these other historical changes in wholeness, glycemic load, and ORAC score also contribute to the pro-inflammatory imbalance characteristic of modern times? Had I inadvertently but fortuitously recreated a modern version of the ancestral diet for myself that had resolved my inflammatory rhinitis? Let's look at each of the measurable characteristics to see how they impact inflammatory predisposition.

The Decline of Wholeness

Wholeness is by far the most important food characteristic in any diet. Wholeness refers to the cellular completeness of a food. If a food retains the same cellular components that it grew with, then it is a whole food. If parts of the food are removed by processing, or if the food is diluted with nonwhole foods, then some degree of wholeness is lost. White flour is about 50 percent whole, because the bran and germ have been milled out. Sugar is less than 1 percent whole since the entire cellular structure of sugar cane has been stripped away. Sugar provides calories and tastes good, but it has nothing left to feed the cellular biochemistry of anyone who eats it.

In order for the reader to visually grasp the impact of wholeness and its decline, I will be using special computer-generated graphics called *NutriCircles©*. This is the software creation of Dr. Donald R. Davis and E. H. Strickland. A working demo can be downloaded from our center's website at the following web address: http://brightspot.org/nutricircles/download.shtml.

NutriCircles do something very special: They allow us to "see" the nutrient composition of almost any food imaginable. When we look at an orange, we see an orange-colored, round piece of fruit. Thanks to Madison Avenue, we probably have the idea that an orange is a good source of vitamin C. We can assume that there are other good nutrients in an orange, but we would be hard-pressed to know which ones and how much of each there are. Trying to compare the nutrient value of an orange with that of a cheeseburger would require hours of searching for data on each. Then, making the actual comparison would be a logistical nightmare.

NutriCircles change all that—dramatically!

Think of NutriCircles as bar graphs in the round. All the bars are actually lines that emanate from the center. Each line represents the content of a nutrient found in the food we are investigating. For example, there would be a vitamin C line for our orange. Better yet, all the U.S. Department of Agriculture's nutrient data for every known nutrient in our orange would also be represented. The result would be a circle with many lines coming out of the center, making it appear like a bicycle wheel with an incomplete set of spokes. Let's focus on the NutriCircle for an orange. (See page 34.)

The outer perimeter of the circle lists the groups of nutrients shown, which include vitamins, trace minerals, major minerals, other nutrients, and amino acids. Inside the perimeter of the circle are abbreviations of these nutrients. Each abbreviation corresponds to a line that represents the amount of that nutrient in an orange.

RDA
Recommended Dietary Allowance, as published by the Food and Nutrition Board of the National Academy of Sciences (USA). Although the RDAs have many limitations, they are the most widely accepted general nutritional standards for U.S. populations.

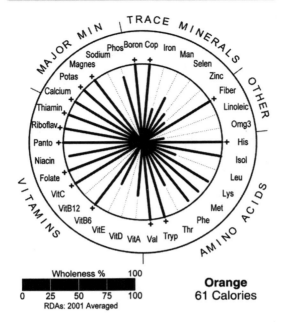

Wholeness %   100

| 0 | 25 | 50 | 75 | 100 |

RDAs: 2001 Averaged

Orange
61 Calories

There is an inner circle in each NutriCircle that closely approximates the RDA for the nutrients listed. If you were to consume 2,500 calories of just oranges in a day, you would get the RDA for those nutrients that reach or exceed the edge of the inner circle. (These bars end in small "plus" signs.) A line that makes it only halfway to that edge indicates that the same amount of oranges contains about half an RDA's worth of that nutrient.

Finally, the small bar graph below each NutriCircle is an actual calculation of the percent of wholeness of the food being investigated. Whole foods always calculate out to 100 percent. This percentage goes down as components of the whole food are lost due to processing or dilution with nonwhole foods.

NutriCircles allow the viewer to assimilate a large amount of nutritional data "in one bite." This gestalt perspective makes it relatively easy to compare the composite nutritional value of various foods. It makes especially evident the devastating effects of nonwhole foods, which will be explained in greater detail in Chapter 8—Our Ancestral Diet.

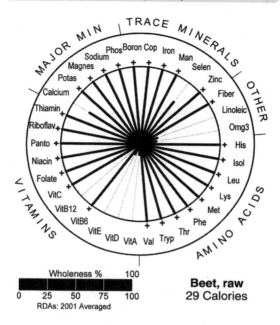

Beet, raw
29 Calories

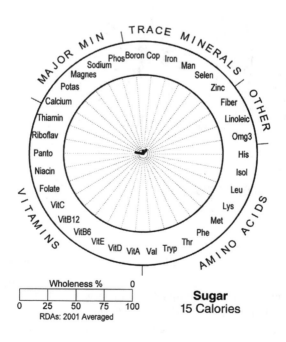

Sugar
15 Calories

Our ancestral diet was 100 percent whole. Primitive humans did not have the ability to alter their foods. Cellular completeness could not be tampered with. With the shift to an agricultural society, butter could be churned, and honeybees were raised, but these and a few other practices resulted in less than a 10 percent reduction in wholeness.

With the industrial age, and the advent of grain mills, the refinement of sugar cane, and the introduction of heavy presses that made vegetable oils, wholeness took a big hit, losing up to 50 to 100 percent or more of nutrients from common sources of calories. (Processed grains, refined sugar, and separated fats make up the "big three" of nonwhole foods.)

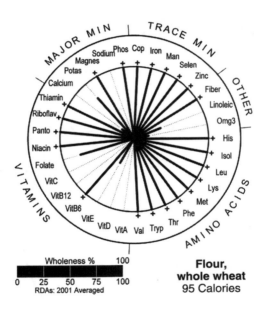

Flour, whole wheat
95 Calories

Around 1950, fast foods emerged as the nutritional paradigm of Western culture. The Happy Meal—burger (grain-fattened beef) on white bun, french fries (predominately vegetable oil), and coke (9 teaspoons of white sugar per standard serving)—is only about 35 percent whole—a very *unhappy* nutritional fact.

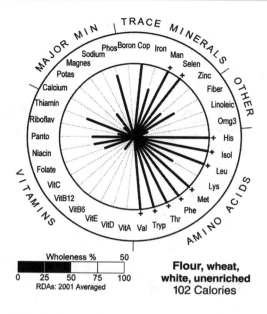

Wholeness %

0   25   50   75   100
RDAs: 2001 Averaged

**Flour, wheat, white, unenriched
102 Calories**

With declining wholeness, nutritional diversity is lost. Fast food alley (aka the American diet) uses the same thirteen foods in 90 percent of its recipes. This increases the probability of adverse food reactions because overconsumption of the same food every day depletes the digestive biochemistry needed to properly break it down and assimilate it. Strawberry jam still retains cooked whole strawberries, but it is only 5 percent whole because the strawberry calories have been diluted 95 percent with the empty calories of sugar. This means that only about 5 percent of the strawberries and the powerful strawberry phytonutrients are still available in each serving of strawberry jam. This is due to a simple dilutional effect of adding nutrient-empty sugar calories to an otherwise excellent nutrient-dense whole food. Dilution creates the delusion that we are eating whole foods when, in reality, we are not.

The colorful fruit and vegetable pigments are excellent antioxidants. The phytonutrient protection of our cells from free-radical damage is largely lost in more modern diets (as reflected in declining ORAC scores). Fiber is also diluted. The loss of fiber sets up

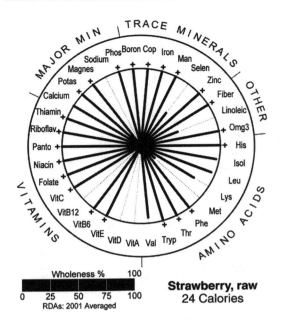

Strawberry, raw
24 Calories

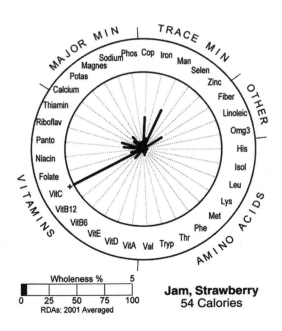

Jam, Strawberry
54 Calories

constipation, but more importantly, it speeds up the absorption of natural sugars in foods. This results in a higher glycemic response and sets the stage for insulin resistance and diabetes.

As depicted in Table 5.2, plant foods were diverse in the hunter-gatherer epoch. This diversity has been almost completely lost in modern times. Eighty percent of Americans fail to eat the "five-a-day" fruits and veggies so necessary for protective phytonutrients, fiber, and low glycemic load. Instead, refined sugar, processed grains, and added bad fats comprise more than 60 percent of modern calories.

TABLE 5.2. CHANGES IN WHAT WE EAT BY EPOCH

Dietary Epoch	Meat	Plant Foods	Grains	Sugar
Hunter-gatherer	Wild	Diverse	None	None
Agricultural	Grass-fed	Gardens	Whole	Rare
Industrial	Grain-fed	Declining	Refined	Common
Fast Food	Feed lots	80% < 5/day	Sweetened	Excess

The Omega-6/Omega-3 Story

The omega-3 fats were abundant in our ancestral diet. Hunter-gatherers hunted grass-fed and bark-fed animals that had a higher omega-3 content in their tissues than grain-fed livestock. Our ancestors had also learned to fish and gather shellfish, which greatly bolstered their EPA intake. High omega-3 foods like fish do so much more than just regulate inflammation; immune function, blood clotting, brain function, and a host of important bodily functions are enhanced with an abundant source of EPA in the diet.

With the addition of grains to the diet thanks to agriculture, the 1:1 omega-6/omega-3 ratio jumped up to 5:1. Grains provide omega-6 calories at the cost of omega-3 sources. Grains were later substituted for grass in feeding livestock, resulting in an even lower omega-3 content in meat.

The industrial era discovery that removing the germ and husks of grains lengthened their storage life inadvertently dropped their percentage of wholeness, wiped out what omega-3 was left, sky-rocketed their glycemic effect, and stripped them of their meager free-radical protection.

Finally, just prior to the fast food epoch, the loss of omega-3 was further compounded with the addition of an "anti-omega-3" compound. Vegetable oil was partially hydrogenated to reduce rancidity. In the process, trans fats were formed in abundance. Result: Consumption of trans fats meant that these fats found their way into cell membranes, disrupting eicosanoid function and further accelerating inflammatory health disorders. Shortly after the introduction of Crisco and hydrogenated margarines, the heart attack rate began to climb precipitously.

My own 17:1 ratio of AA/EPA back in 2001 (see Chapter 4) was typical of the 20:1 omega-6/omega-3 ratio estimated to represent the fast food epoch. Convenience foods had made their way into our home. Trans fats were lurking in baked goods, microwave popcorn, and even whole-grain bread. It was in 2002 that my cytotoxic food-sensitivity test showed that I adversely reacted to wheat. I began to eliminate baked goods from my diet. This lowering of omega-6 fat intake coincided with raising my intake of pharmaceutical-grade omega-3 supplements. These behavioral changes helped me to drop my AA/EPA ratio to 5:1.

Glycemic Chaos

The *glycemic index* (GI) for any food is calculated by giving volunteers enough of a test food to equal 50 grams of carbohydrate for that food. Blood sugar levels are then drawn like a glucose tolerance test. The results are compared to the subject's glucose control test, and expressed as a percentage—the area under the test food's curve divided by the area under their glucose curve. For example, 120 grams of watermelon carbohydrate produces a curve about 72 percent of the control glucose curve. Glycemic load is the glycemic index divided by 100 multiplied by its available carbohydrate content (that is, carbohydrates minus fiber) in grams. Use serving size in grams for calculating the glycemic index. Watermelon's glycemic index is pretty high, about 72. According to the calculations by the people at the University of Sydney's Human Nutrition Unit, in a serving of 120 grams of watermelon, there are 6 grams of available carbohydrate per serving so its glycemic load is pretty low—$72 \div 100 \times 6 = 4.32$, rounded to 4.

The American Diabetic Association's Public Relation Team gives the following examples to help you visualize standard serving sizes:

- Three ounces of cooked meat, fish, or poultry is the size of a deck of cards.

- Two tablespoons of peanut butter is the size of a golf ball.

- A medium piece of fruit looks like a baseball.

- A medium bagel is the size of a hockey puck.

- One ounce of cheese is the size of four dice.

- A small baked potato is the size of a computer mouse.

- The serving size for raw vegetables, yogurt, and fruit is one cup—which fits into an average woman's hand.

The result gives you a good idea of just how much insulin it will take to process the carbohydrates in a serving of carrots.

Carrots are a whole food like the food our ancestors ate from a diverse array of plant-derived foods. Most of these ancestral foods were highly colorful and had very low GLs. Whole grains have a higher GL. Refined grains have an even higher GL. Consuming sugary soda pop (very high GL) along with french fries (high GL) and burgers on white bread (moderately high GL), all team up together to produce a very high glycemic load. In a fast food society, insulin levels run high on an almost continuous basis. High GL eating sets the stage for high insulin levels, metabolic syndrome, diabetes, heart disease, and a host of severe degenerative illnesses.

High insulin levels favor the production of arachidonic acid (AA). The enzyme responsible for taking omega-6 fats and converting them into the pro-inflammatory AA is stimulated by insulin. Choosing a low glycemic diet like that of our ancestors will reduce AA production. This step, in combination with an increased intake of ocean fish and omega-3 supplements, favorably lowers the AA/EPA ratio.

When I found that I was sensitive to wheat, I eliminated all bread and grains from my diet. About that same time I started giving Atkins lectures. I eliminated sugar and snacks made with hydrogenated oils. I emphasized grass-fed beef and ate more ocean fish. My diet became almost 100 percent whole. My omega-3 intake increased dramatically. The glycemic index of my foods was very low. The cumulative ORAC Score (see discussion below) of my foods skyrocketed with my decision to have some kind of berry every day. (Blueberries and other berries are the ORAC All Stars!)

Oxygen Radical Absorbance Capacity

Researchers at the USDA's Human Nutrition Research Center at Tufts University in Boston developed a method of analyzing individual foods for their antioxidant capacity. Then another USDA scientist, Dr. Guohua Cao, blended some samples of specified foods and used the pulp and extract to reveal the food's "total antioxidant capacity or power." The procedure is now referred to as ORAC (Oxygen Radical Absorbance Capacity).

Our ancestral diet was rich in diversity and quantity of plant-based foods. The more colorful varieties of plant foods were sure to attract our ancestors' attention. The darker and richer the color pigments, the higher the free-radical-absorbing capacity. (See Table 5.3—Top Antioxidant Foods.)

With the advent of agriculture, gathering was limited to what grew in the garden. Some of the diver-

TABLE 5.3. TOP ANTIOXIDANT FOODS— ORAC UNITS PER 100 GRAMS			
Fruits	**ORAC**	**Veggies**	**ORAC**
Prunes	5,770	Kale	1,770
Raisins	2,830	Spinach	1,260
Blueberries	2,400	Brussels sprouts	980
Blackberries	2,036	Alfalfa sprouts	930
Strawberries	1,540	Broccoli	890
Raspberries	1,220	Beets	840
Plums	949	Red Peppers	710
Oranges	750	Onions	450
Red Grapes	739	Corn	400
Cherries	670	Eggplant	390

(Note: If this chart was expressed in ORAC units *per serving* prunes and raisins would not top the list. Removing water from plums and grapes simply gives you prunes and raisins; it does not magically impart a greater ORAC score. The dehydrating process simply *concentrates* the antioxidants in these two foods.)

sity was lost. Industrial cultures were even further removed from wild plants and civilized gardens. Fruits and veggies had to be shipped at a premium to industrial centers with loss of variety and quality. In the fast food era, vegetables are a mere garnishing. Fruits are often limited to the picture of the fruit flavoring on the beverage container.

This extreme loss of antioxidant power favors the destructive effect of chronic inflammation. White blood cells release tissue-destructive lysozymes, which generate excessive free radicals. Without the protective power of high ORAC foods, these free radicals roam unchecked, damaging cell membranes, DNA, and a host of important cellular structures. Over time, this adds greatly to the slow degenerative nature of chronic low-grade inflammation.

Four Key Characteristics of Our Ancestral Diet

To summarize, our ancestral diet provided four key

benefits that have generally been lost in the modern "civilized" diet.

- **Whole foods**, rich in antioxidants, protect cells from excess lysozymal, free-radical formation. Whole foods are also rich in fiber, which lowers their glycemic index. Eliminating nonwhole foods such as sugar and white flour further enhances these benefits.

- **A low omega-6/omega-3 ratio (AA/EPA)** lowers the pro-inflammatory AA precursor and raises the anti-inflammatory EPA regulation.

- **A low glycemic index** keeps insulin levels low and results in lower conversion of omega-6 to pro-inflammatory eicosanoids. By avoiding diabetes, fewer *advanced glycation end products* (AGEs) are formed. These end products are extremely potent free radicals that only add to the damage being done by excessive lysozyme-generated free radicals.

- **High ORAC foods** absorb free radicals and limit the degenerative "injury" which acts to perpetuate the excessive inflammatory triggering that occurs in chronic inflammation.

Our ancestral diet naturally and automatically provided humans with these key dietary regulators of inflammation. The pro-inflammatory dietary shifts described in this chapter demonstrate that this nutritional "safety net" has badly eroded. We can no longer assume that modern foods will protect us from excessive inflammation. The rapid rise in chronic inflammatory/degenerative illness in modern times is clear evidence of this.

In order to derive the built-in regulation of inflammation provided by our ancestral diet, modern humans must go out of their way to understand and regularly choose whole foods. Ocean seafood and grass- and plant-fed animals along with high-quality fish oil supplements will normalize one's omega-6/omega-3 ratio. Colorful plant-based foods are low glycemic and high ORAC and should be consumed in abundant diversity in one's diet.

I was able to recreate the ancestral diet and control my allergic rhinitis. You can do the same to control *your* chronic inflammation. No matter what "-itis" you are struggling with, recreating the ancestral diet through proper food selection and dietary supplementation will help you overcome your pro-inflammatory predisposition and restore balance to your wonderful inflammatory system.

CHAPTER 6

MOUTH/HEART INFLAMMATION

Paula's Story

Paula was sixteen when her dentist diagnosed *trench mouth*. Her gums were sore and bleeding. The dentist prescribed an antibiotic. A few days later the pain eased and the active bleeding stopped. Her gums remained inflamed and still bled from time to time.

Paula had begun smoking two years earlier. Both her parents smoked, so she didn't think of it as a bad habit. The dentist told her that the smoking probably contributed to her trench mouth. What he didn't know was that the trench mouth and the smoking together would contribute to Paula's heart disease almost forty years later.

Periodontal Disease

Trench mouth is a severe form of periodontal disease. Periodontal disease is also called gingivitis. The suffix "-itis" indicates *inflammation of the gingiva* or gums surrounding the teeth. Not surprisingly, gingivitis elevates CRP. Smoking also elevates CRP. Even a half-a-pack a day smoker is *three times* more likely to develop gingivitis. Gingivitis and smoking together amplify the body's inflammatory response.

Even when not painful and swollen, inflamed gums are known to harbor infection. A bacterium called *Chlamydia pneumoniae* has been found living in atherosclerotic plaque. Could there be a link between smoking, inflamed and infected gums, and the development of artery disease? In 1997, J. B. Muhlestein published a study that demonstrated a causal relationship.

Muhlestein purposefully infected rabbits with chlamydia and found that the development of plaque in their arteries was accelerated. Treating the rabbits with an antibiotic prevented the plaque development. We can only presume that had Muhlestein been able to teach the rabbits to smoke, their arterial plaque might have developed even faster.

Syndrome X

By the time Paula was fifty years old, her blood pressure started to run high. A cosmetologist, she often felt hurried to stay on schedule. To manage her stress, she turned to eating. As a child she rarely ate sweets, but times had changed and so had her taste buds. She craved sugary sweets: cookies, pies, and cakes. Her missed meals were supplanted with high-carbohydrate snack foods. The pounds began to pile up on Paula. Her blood sugar levels were okay in spite of a diabetic heritage on her paternal side. Her blood triglycerides did not fare so well; they skyrocketed to 429!

A hysterectomy in her middle forties meant that she needed to take Premarin, an estrogen replacement pill. Estrogen tends to destabilize blood sugar levels, stimulate hunger, and add more pounds. Five feet five, Paula peaked at 182 pounds. Paula's cholesterol was more than 300 even before she turned thirty. When she came to me in 1992, at age forty-four, her total cholesterol topped 330.

In 1992, I was unaware of the fine work of Stanford professor Dr. Gerald M. Reaven who had identified a constellation of high-risk symptoms. Dr. Reaven observed that (1) abdominal obesity, (2) high blood pressure, (3) glucose intolerance, and (4) abnormal blood lipids often occurred together. He coined the name *Syndrome X*, now also known as *metabolic syndrome*. Researchers estimate that nearly half of all Americans can now be diagnosed with Syndrome X! Paula was one of them.

Each of the individual components of Syndrome X increases the risk of developing diabetes and heart disease. Combining two or more of these risk factors has a cumulative effect on the risk of developing diabetes, having a heart attack, or both. To make matters worse, Paula had two more red flags: an elevated homocysteine level and sky-high lipoprotein (a).

The Genesis of Plaque

Homocysteine is a metabolite of the amino acid methionine. In the absence of adequate folic acid, and vitamins B_6 and B_{12}, homocysteine cannot be properly metabolized. It accumulates in the bloodstream, becoming toxic to the lining of arteries. It causes a type of chemical injury, and injuries trigger cytokines. As you recall, cytokines will loosen the junctions between the endothelial cells of the injured artery. White blood cells move through these gaps into the arterial wall. Then more cytokines are released that signal the white cells to change into debris-eating macrophages.

Metabolite
The biochemical result or product of a metabolic pathway necessary to sustain the life of cells.

If any cholesterol has accumulated in the artery, especially in an oxidized form of cholesterol called *LDL cholesterol,* it is devoured by the macrophages. Soon the macrophages become loaded with fat. Researchers call these "obese" cells *foam cells.*

Foam cells secrete additional pro-inflammatory substances that set up a chronic triggering of the process over and over again. This is precisely how acute arterial inflammation grinds into a chronic phase. Repeatedly, low-grade damage to the muscle cells in the arterial walls results in the deposition of collagen and lipoproteins. Plaque forms. The artery starts to narrow as fatty streaks appear. The plaque itself becomes fertile ground for infection with chlamydia from infected gums. This further stimulates the inflammatory cascade.

These silent moments of inflammation incubate for decades. Then, in one fateful moment, a tiny rupture occurs in the plaque. Clot formation is triggered. Blood flow is blocked. Oxygen cannot be delivered to highly metabolic cardiac cells. Within minutes, chest pains ensue.

Men often have the classic exertional heaviness in their chest. Rest will not relieve it. In women, the symptoms are menacingly vague: maybe sudden, deep fatigue or feeling short of breath. If undiagnosed, the heart attack victim is at grave risk for fatal arrhythmias.

Predicting a Heart Attack

Paula had her first CRP test at age fifty-four. It was 6.2 milligrams per liter, more than double the highest risk for potential heart attack. Dr. Paul Ridker published several studies on CRP in the *New England Journal of Medicine* from 1997 to 2002. Looking at cholesterol and CRP in 28,263 women, Dr. Ridker found that CRP predicted cardiac risk *four times better* than LDL cholesterol did. Paula's high CRP would have meant that she was in grave danger. Unfortunately the danger had already struck. I had drawn her CRP almost three months after her heart attack.

Women have atypical symptoms of heart disease. The medical model of acute coronary syndrome was based on male symptomatology. Paula never had chest pain. The shoulder pain she had when she exerted herself was relieved by rest. Her doctor did not suspect heart disease. He sent her for an MRI of her shoulder and mistakenly diagnosed *tendonitis*. The doctor was looking for inflammation in the wrong place.

After several months of progressively increasing shoulder pain, Paula's left jaw area began to hurt with exertion. One day while walking the jaw pain became excruciating and was not relieved by rest. Paula was rushed to the emergency room. Tests showed her left coronary artery was 90 percent blocked; the right one was 50 percent blocked. Her cardiologist positioned a medicated stent into her left coronary, hoping to restore normal blood flow. Fortunately, Paula suffered only minimal damage to her heart muscle.

The Road to Recovery

Paula had quit smoking a few years before her heart attack. Now she was more than ready to tackle her diet. Her cardiologist put her on medications to control her blood pressure and thin her blood. He also started her on a statin drug to lower her cholesterol. She could not continue it due to severe muscle aches and elevated liver enzymes. Instead, Paula took the cholesterol-lowering vitamin niacin, a high-potency multivitamin, and fish oil.

Thirteen years before her heart attack, Paula had the fatty acids test done at our center laboratory. Her profile measured levels of omega-3 and omega-6 fatty acids, along with levels of saturated and monounsaturated fatty acids. Her low eicosapentaenoic omega-3 level stood out. It was in just the 10th percentile. Paula was low in the oil best derived from fish, and Paula hated fish.

Eight months after her heart attack, she was taking fish oil capsules, and her CRP had dropped from 6.2 to 3.7 milligrams per liter. (See Table 6.1.) One year later, by adding a regular walking program and following a carbohydrate-controlled, whole foods diet together with her fish oil capsules, she had lowered her CRP to 0.9 milligrams per liter! Two years after her heart attack, Paula had dropped her weight from 182 to 143 pounds and was able to discontinue her blood pressure medications. With careful blood nutrient testing, we developed Paula's supplement program.

TABLE 6.1. PAULA'S SUPPLEMENT PROGRAM

Supplement	Dose	Reason for taking
Ester C	500 mg	Antioxidant
Folic acid	1,600 mg	To lower homocysteine
Fish oil caps	3,000 mg	Anti-inflammatory, and more
Coenzyme Q_{10}	100 mg	Antioxidant that improves cellular-energy production
Niacin	1,000 mg	Cholesterol control, raises HDL
Red yeast rice	1,200 mg	Natural source statin analogs
Vitamin E	800 IU	Fat soluble antioxidant, lowers CRP
Pantothenic acid	500 mg	Adrenal and joint support
Policosanol	10 mg	Cholesterol control
USP thyroid	90 mg	Metabolism
Aspirin	325 mg	Antiplatelet aggregation
DHEA	5 mg	Low blood levels, blood sugar regulator

Mouth-to-Mouth Resuscitation

After her heart attack, Paula took charge of her health (and her mouth!). She quit smoking. She embraced the diet of our ancestors. She exercised. She lost weight. Fish oil supplements lowered the hidden inflammation in her body. Antioxidant supplements slowed oxidative damage. Other supplements enhanced her nutritional wholeness. These lifestyle changes have lowered her risk for further arterial damage.

Paula is taking a college class in oral communication. She is required to make a major presentation for her final grade. She wants to tell the story of her heart disease. She observes the lifestyles of the younger college students in her class. Some are smoking. Some are buying junk food. Undoubtedly, some have gingivitis and are unaware of its relationship to heart disease.

Paula hopes that someone listening will learn from her experience. Low-grade, systemic inflammation is silent and hidden. Biochemical clues, if measured, can alert you to its sinister presence. A CRP must be included as part of a complete cardiovascular risk assessment, along with measurement of the homocysteine level, and of the levels of lipoprotein (a), fasting blood sugar, and LDL and HDL cholesterol. Monitor your blood pressure, abdominal girth, and weight. Rising levels can alert you to hidden arterial damage, plaque formation, and the risk of sudden blockage and heart attack. For 50 percent of heart disease suffers, sudden death is the first indication of the illness!

Paula wants to be a "human cytokine." She wants to signal a warning to other people: Wake up! Your arteries are being silently damaged as we speak! Your only defense is informed action. Measure your risk factors! Heed your numbers! The risk is real! Heart disease can be prevented. You can disarm America's number-one killer. Its weapon is *undetected, low-grade, systemic inflammation.* You have the power to recognize and disarm it. Use it!

CHAPTER 7

GUT/JOINT INFLAMMATION

Gene's Story

Gene was looking forward to his retirement. He had been saving two old cars: a '54 Chevy that needed to be customized and a '77 Jaguar that needed refurbishing. He had his shop all ready to go.

But elevated PSA tests (*prostatic surface antigen* is a marker for possible prostate cancer) kept getting in the way. Two previous prostate biopsies for cancer were negative, but this last one had found it. Each biopsy had been followed with a round of antibiotics to prevent secondary infection.

The doctors told Gene he needed a total body CT scan and a colonoscopy to make sure the cancer had not spread. His intestines were flushed with a diarrhea-causing electrolyte solution. Everything tested okay. He was ready for an abdominal radical prostatectomy. Powerful intravenous antibiotics were given post-op. Gene pulled through fine and was sent home on two weeks of oral antibiotics. He was on the road to recovery, eager to get to working on his show cars.

Then the pain started with a vengeance.

Rheumatoid Arthritis

Severe joint pains in his hands and wrists broke the previously reliable pattern of his sleep. The swelling and awful aching was like nothing Gene had ever experienced before. Ice packs were required just to get through the evenings and to get to sleep. His family doctor referred Gene to a rheumatologist (a specialist in arthritis and other inflammatory conditions). He confirmed Gene's worst fear: he had rheumatoid arthritis (RA).

RA is nothing short of an all-out assault by the body's white blood cells on selected joints. One in fifty Americans suffer with RA. As common as it is, the cause is unknown. RA demonstrates all five of the classic signs of acute inflammation: pain, swelling, heat, redness, and loss of function. But RA inflammation is chronic. As the disease progresses in time, joints are literally destroyed by the chemical byproducts of inflammation. Joint replacement surgery is all too common.

RA extends beyond joints into low-grade systemic inflammation. General fatigue, anemia, depression, heart symptoms, blood vessel inflammation, and even lung involvement are part of the disease's systemic spread.

Gene's rheumatologist suggested Plaquenil to get control of his runaway pain. Curiously, Plaquenil is an antimalarial drug. In the RA setting, it is considered a DMARD—a disease-modifying antirheumatic drug. The inflammation is quelled for reasons that are unclear. Unfortunately, a damaging side effect can occur in the retina. Gene went to his ophthalmologist to get his opinion on Plaquenil. The physician advised staying off the drug for as long as possible.

Increased Intestinal Permeability

Rheumatologists treat RA with rather powerful pharmaceutical weapons. NSAIDs are the mainstay of therapy. As powerful and potentially dangerous as they are, NSAIDs are often no match for severe RA.

NSAIDs
Nonsteroidal anti-inflammatory drugs; inhibitors of the COX pro-inflammatory enzymes.

Gene tried ibuprofen—800 milligrams, one to three times daily. It helped him to get by, but he felt like it was only covering up the pain without treating the underlying cause of the persistent joint inflammation. Paradoxically, ibuprofen has been shown to cause inflammation in the stomach and intestinal lining. RA subjects in a *Lancet* study taking NSAIDs were found to have increased *intestinal permeability*.

Aging alone has been shown to increase the intestinal absorption of large molecules. Proteins are large molecules composed of long chains of amino acids. Digestive enzymes sever these chains into smaller peptide snippets. The peptides are digested into individual amino acids prior to absorption.

Immune Complexes

With increased intestinal permeability, the larger peptide molecules are absorbed *prematurely*. These peptides are too large for cells to utilize. The immune system then treats the peptides as foreign proteins. Antibodies are made which latch on to multiple peptides and result in a clumping phenomenon. These clumps are called *immune complexes*. White blood cells phagocytize (engulf and destroy) these complexes.

This is all well and good except for one major issue: cytokines. Once you are sensitized to protein-containing food, consuming that food triggers antibody formation and the release of cytokines. Antibodies are made by *lymphocytes*—specialized immune cells that remember you have previously reacted to a partially digested protein, such as wheat gluten. If you are one of the estimated 50 percent of the American population that has a partial (and often silent) sensitivity to wheat gluten, your inflammatory system will react to gluten time and time again. Pro-inflammatory cytokines will build up in your bloodstream.

Food Addictions

As part of the cytokine alarm signal, there is a systemic response to the "stress" of gluten exposure. This includes adrenaline release, endorphin production, and a small burst of cortisol production by the adrenals to help you adapt. These adaptive molecules are made by the adrenal glands and brain. Though short-lived, this adaptive burst feels good. It wakes you up, reduces your pain, and even reshuffles your neurotransmitters in a favorable way. As a result, you go for wheat again and again, until you are thoroughly "addicted" to this cytokine-induced response to any of the many wheat products available. This is how "cookie-monsters" are created.

Sounds innocent enough. However, the immune complexes that are formed can get stuck in the basement membranes of almost any organ. Should that organ be the capsule that lines your finger and wrist joints, the net result will be arthritis symptoms in your hands, like Gene's. White blood cells attack the immune complexes. The white cells are filled with tiny organelles called *lysosomes*.

Lysozymes

When a white cell engulfs bacteria or immune complexes or cellular debris of any sort, these lysosomes attach themselves to the engulfed object. Lysosomal enzymes called *lysozymes* are released in an attempt to break down and digest the object. This approach works very well in acute inflammation. Redness, swelling, and pain are signs that the white blood cells have released their lysozymes, and the battle to disinfect and clean up the injury zone is well under way.

Lysozymes
Enzymes made by special white blood cells called macrophages; they are used to digest damaged tissues, infecting organisms, or foreign proteins.

With immune complexes that have formed from wheat gluten or other sensitive foods, the battle never ends. The protein antigen shows up over and over, every day, often several times a day if you crave wheat at every meal and every snack. Cytokines are repeatedly triggered. More white blood cells arrive. More lysozymes are released. Lysozymes work by creating free radicals to attack the foreign proteins. With chronic inflammation, free-radical formation becomes uncontrolled. Free-radical damage spills over into healthy tissues. Over time, the connective tissue that is the structural backbone of the joint begins to erode. Rheumatologists call this process *degenerative* arthritis.

The process never completes itself because food

addictions make it seem like you cannot live without the addictive food. You believe that food makes you feel better! (Thanks to adrenaline, endorphins, and cortisol.) Meanwhile, a barrage of immune complexes flood affected joints. Inflammation rages like an out-of-control forest fire. You and your doctor pour on the NSAIDs in a desperate attempt to put out the inflammatory fire.

In Gene, this process showed up as RA. This same sequence of events can cause any one of many chronic inflammatory syndromes: colitis, dermatitis, vasculitis, lupus, and gastritis—it just depends on where the immune complexes get stuck, based upon your genetic susceptibility or prior injury.

The Cytotoxic Test

When Gene came to see me, we performed a comprehensive laboratory evaluation. There is one blood test we do on every arthritis patient: the cytotoxic test. While shunned by conventional rheumatologists, when correctly done, the cytotoxic test provides invaluable information about food sensitivities. There are food elimination protocols to help patients determine their sensitive foods, but they are time-consuming and can be difficult to stick with. A fasting blood sample is all that is needed for the cytotoxic to reveal inflammatory food triggers.

Gene's cytotoxic was unlike any I had previously seen. The cytotoxic test tests ninety common *food antigens*. Typically 20 to 30 percent will be reactive in the average American. In Gene, more than 80 percent of the food antigens tested were reactive! I told Gene that his gut was highly inflamed and highly permeable to reactive peptides.

What caused this in Gene? Certainly the ibuprofen was partly to blame, but many patients on NSAIDs do not have nearly as intense a cytotoxic response as Gene. Was there another explanation?

Candida Overgrowth

Because of Gene's history of multiple rounds of antibiotics following his biopsies and prostate surgery, I tested his candida antibody titers. Candida is a common fungal organism known as a commensurate organism in the lining of the gut. In healthy individuals, small numbers of candida live harmlessly among the more than 100 trillion friendly bacteria that inhabit the lining of our intestines and colon.

With multiple rounds of antibiotics, this delicate gut ecology gets disrupted. The antibiotics kill off a large segment of the friendly lactobacillus, thus allowing the *overgrowth* of the candida species. This is analogous to overspraying your lawn with weed killer. A large part of the good grass is knocked out, which allows the crabgrass or other weeds to overgrow.

Gene's candida antibody titers were very high, much higher than an individual who has the normal exposure to candida. This indicated that his immune system was trying to control the overgrowth of yeast, but had not yet succeeded. Candida exists in two basic forms: budding yeast and the fungal form with penetrating hyphae. The penetrating hyphae burrow into the endothelial lining of the gut, making it more permeable. Candida overgrowth is almost always associated with heightened food sensitivities.

Gene's CRP reflected his inflammatory state, though not as high as is commonly seen in RA. His CRP was 4.4 milligrams per liter. His AA/ EPA ratio (omega 6/omega 3) was 13.77:0.61 giving him a 27:1 pro-inflammatory predisposition. Lowering this ratio would lower Gene's predisposition to inflammation. He was also quite low in GLA, which added to his pro-inflammatory tendencies.

Gene's Treatment Plan

The testing mentioned above was done as part of Gene's first appointment at the center. Only one supplement was prescribed then: *nattokinase*. Nattokinase is an enzyme derived from fermented soy. It has the unique ability to break down fibrin that has accumulated in the bloodstream. Chronically ill patients often complain of poor circulation. The triggering of fibrin formation in the blood causes increased blood viscosity and decreased circulation through certain capillary beds in afflicted individuals.

At Gene's second appointment we reviewed his lab work. I was struck with Gene's dramatic cytotoxic results. We discussed the leaky gut syndrome. To heal the gut I suggested he take an undenatured (unheated) whey protein product to serve as a precursor to *glutathione*. Glutathione is a small protein molecule composed of the three amino acids: cysteine, glycine, and glutamic acid. Glutathione is often referred to as the body's master antioxidant. In addition, glutathione regulates immune function and acts as a crucial step in liver detoxification pathways. Glutathione can be purchased as a supplement, but is poorly absorbed. The stomach digests this protein before much can be absorbed. Undenatured whey contains the three constituent amino acids of glutathione in abundance. Cells that line the gut get first pick of these aminos and can then synthesize glutathione. After the three aminos are absorbed, their first stop is the liver, where glutathione plays a crucial role in detoxification.

In addition to the whey, I prescribed a potent acidophilus combination to replenish the friendly flora of the gut lining. Candida is described as an opportunistic organism. All the antibiotics that Gene had taken around the time of his biopsies and surgeries had wiped out a significant portion of the friendly gut flora, thus allowing candida to overgrow in abundance. Candida released metabolic waste products that acted as toxins to the lining of the gut and the liver. Candida hyphae burrowed into the gut making it even more inflamed and permeable.

Here's how I explained Gene's large number of sensitive foods: Stress had weakened his immune system; antibiotics had disrupted his gut flora; candida had overgrown and caused increased gut permeability; food proteins were absorbed in a partially digested state called peptides; the peptides acted as antigens and triggered antibody formation; the antibodies attached to the peptides; immune complexes formed in the bloodstream; finally, these complexes got stuck in the basement membranes of Gene's joints. Gene's inflamed gut and adverse food reactions led to his diagnosis of RA.

Two other treatments were recommended at that appointment: (1) an EPA-containing fish oil supplement that also contained borage oil, a good source of GLA. I recommended he take two at breakfast and two at supper; (2) 3 teaspoons of MSM powder (organic sulfur to help repair connective tissue) in a quart of water that he was to drink throughout the day as a natural anti-inflammatory strategy. I asked Gene to return in one month to assess his progress.

"I'm Well"

One month later, Gene showed up for his third appointment. When I walked into the exam room I greeted Gene and his wife Karen, and asked Gene how he was doing. "I'm well," was his nonchalant reply. "What about all that pain?" I asked. He said the pain was almost gone. I told him he needed to be serious. He *was* serious! The pain had started in his fingers, hands, and wrists. Then it had moved into his hips and knees. Now the pain had left his hands and fingers, and was currently leaving his hips and knees. Since his previous appointment one month ago he had taken only two of the 200-milligram ibuprofens—and that was for other reasons!

Four months later, the pain relief was holding. Gene had learned which foods he could get away with, and which he had to either completely avoid or use infrequently. He was eating a lot of berries and frozen grapes. He had to avoid peanuts and shellfish completely. There were few fried foods left on their menu.

Eighteen months after his initial treatment at the center, Gene remains pain free and active. During this time period he pulled the engine from that '77 Jag, rebuilt it, and put it back in himself! He painted the car bright yellow and sold it for a nifty profit. He's still working on the Chevy.

Gene always knew he would get better. He believed in the power of a positive attitude. But attitude alone is usually not enough. He takes his fatty acids and a few other supplements. He focuses on whole foods. He loves his wife and his cars.

He knows that he can do anything he wants to do and needs to do "with energy and enthusiasm." He reached this point by being willing to look for the underlying causes of his rampant inflammation. As a colearner he found those causes, corrected them, and regained his good health, his great attitude, and the freedom to do what he wants!

CHAPTER 8

OUR ANCESTRAL DIET

Our ancestors had no choice; they had to eat whole foods.

Food is life. All foods were once alive. Foods are composed of or made from cells. Cells contain special chemicals that maintain life. The foods we eat give us the cellular biochemicals we need to sustain the lives of our own cells.

The Cellular Basis of Whole Foods

All living things—plants, animals, fungi, and algae—consist of cells. Cells require a metabolism to live. Their metabolic chemistry is amazingly similar to our own. We all share the same need for fats, proteins, and carbohydrates. Our micronutrient needs parallel the micronutrient needs of the cells that comprise our food. In essence, this defines food. Food is food because of this amazing biochemical unity that exists at the cellular level of all life on this planet.

Our cells and organs are composed of basic biochemicals. Of these there are more than forty known essential nutrients, including ten essential amino acids, two essential fatty acids, thirteen or so vitamins, more than fifteen minerals, and several other essential nutrients that must be adequately derived from our diet or taken as supplements in order to maintain the cellular life. Because all foods are cellular in origin (milk is not a cellular food, though it is derived directly from cells and serves as a food for growing infants), we derive these essential nutrients from them. It is automatic, *if our food's wholeness is retained*!

Eat a Variety of Whole Foods

Whole foods are not the same in their nutrient mix. Different organisms use different arrays of nutrients for different adaptive functions. Fish cells have a different adaptive challenge than walnut cells. Although fish cells and walnut cells both contain omega-3 fats, fish cells have a much higher content. Plankton are tiny organisms rich in omega-3 fats. The ocean food chain starts with plankton. The higher omega-3 content of fish cells allows fish to adapt to a different living environment than walnuts do.

Fruits, though not known as protein foods, do require amino acids for their cellular livelihood. Looking at the NutriCircle of an orange, it might be surprising to learn that twenty out of thirty-four essential nutrients shown are present in RDA-adequate amounts in an orange. Looking at amino acids in particular, it is interesting to note that an "orangetarian" would probably not become protein deficient. The lack of omega-3 in oranges would cause omega-3 deficiency symptoms and health consequences would eventually ensue.

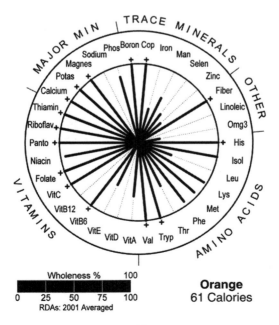

Orange
61 Calories

Adding to the twenty adequate nutrients, another ten of these essential nutrients are present in oranges, but in sub-RDA amounts. With twenty out of thirty-four essential nutrients being present in oranges, our hypothetical "orangetarian" would live fairly well on this particular whole food.

"Eggetarians" would do even better. (Compare the NutriCircles for oranges and eggs.) Almost all of the nutrients present in eggs reach adequate RDA status. By eating a variety of whole foods the strengths of one fill in the weaknesses of another.

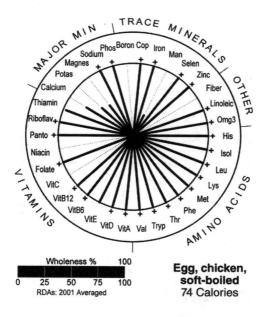

Wholeness %				100
0	25	50	75	100

RDAs: 2001 Averaged

Egg, chicken, soft-boiled
74 Calories

The Biochemical Unity of Life

Our ancestors lived off of this great biochemical unity of life. All living creatures live off it as well. By eating whole foods that retain their cellular structure, our preagricultural ancestors consumed an adequate array of essential nutrients. Whole foods allowed them to survive and thrive.

The last several millennia have witnessed a drastic change in our ancestral diet. Agricultural technology has allowed mankind to reduce whole foods to food parts. The dismantlement of whole foods into food parts has resulted in the wholesale consumption of nonwhole foods. Dr. Don Davis, a chemist and student of the late great whole foods advocate, Dr. Roger Williams, calls these nonwhole foods *dismembered foods*. *Dismembered foods now make up more than half of the modern American diet!*

The Evolution of the Orange

One of the great pleasures in life is to get a big fresh orange and hand peel it. The aroma alone is worth the effort. Then you get to eat it slice by slice. Let's look at the NutriCircle of a whole orange again.

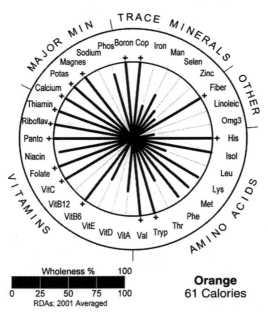

Orange
61 Calories

In the NutriCircle of the whole orange you can see that one serving is sixty-one calories. The outer circle is divided into amino acids, vitamins, major minerals, trace minerals, and other nutrients, with all of the individual nutrients labeled with abbreviations. The inner circle represents the percent of one RDA for each nutrient listed if you consumed 2,500 calories worth of the food depicted, in this case, oranges. Below and to the left is a bar graph calculation of the wholeness of the food expressed as a percentage.

(See pages 32–34 for a more complete explanation of how to read a NutriCircle graphic.)

What happens if you process whole oranges just a bit? What if you were to make frozen canned orange juice out of them? How would that change the NutriCircle?

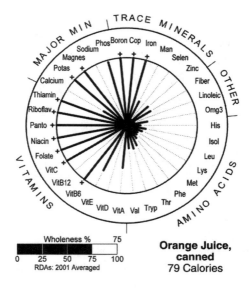

Wholeness % 75

0   25   50   75   100
RDAs: 2001 Averaged

Orange Juice, canned
79 Calories

Notice right away how the wholeness dropped 25 percent. That's because some rind and some fiber was lost in the juicing process. Notice how amino acids have dropped out. Overall the NutriCircle is not as well filled out as the orange NutriCircle.

What about shifting now to an orange drink that you can buy at the grocery store—"with 200 percent of the daily requirement of vitamin C added!"?(See page 66.)

You will immediately notice that almost all of the previous nutrients are now missing. Wholeness has dropped to a miserable 5 percent. The manufacturer has added the only nutrients available in this "food." Otherwise it is just sugar water with a few vitamins and some orange coloring. In spite of this terrible showing, this product is purchased everywhere by mothers thinking they are giving their kids something healthy and palatable.

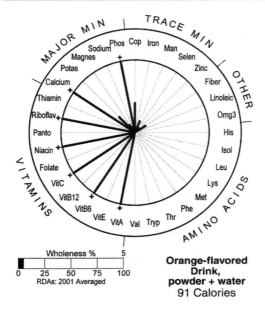

Orange-flavored Drink, powder + water
91 Calories

Now we take the final step in the evolution of the orange: orange soda pop. You can buy it almost anywhere. Pop machines are ubiquitous. Most of the orange soda pop companies have put a nice picture of an orange on the can.

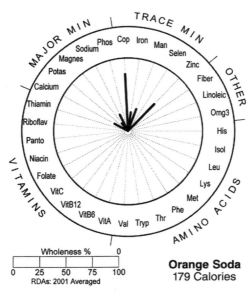

Orange Soda
179 Calories

What you see is what you get: *nada!* Orange soda is just sugar, fizzy water, and orange coloring. This NutriCircle is nearly identical to the one for sugar on page 35. It depicts the nutritional devastation of non-whole foods. You buy a picture of an orange on a can. Your cells get nothing!

When the whole orange is traded for a can of orange soda, look what happens:

- the fiber and pulp have been removed

- the colorful and health-protective phytonutrients are gone (potentially toxic artificial coloring has been added)

- ninety-nine percent of *all* nutrients are now missing

- more than 100 calories of pure sugar calories are consumed

- the body is forced to draw upon nutrient reserves to process the nutrient-empty sugar calories

- over time, the addictive habit of sugar and other dismembered foods greatly depletes nutrient reserves

- the high sugar content is rapidly absorbed, creating a glucose spike and an insulin surge (hyperinsulinemia) that inexorably leads to insulin resistance and diabetes (sugar is the reference food used to define *high glycemic index*)

Nonwhole foods lead to the overconsumption of empty or near-empty calories. The United States probably leads the world in the consumption of nonwhole foods. It is no coincidence that the United States is also the world leader in obesity, diabetes, heart disease, and a long list of chronic inflammatory diseases and degenerative disorders.

Nonwhole Foods

There are four categories of nonwhole foods: refined sugars, processed grains, separated and altered fats, and alcohol. Rarely are these foods eaten "straight."

There are few among us who would take a sugar bowl and spoon sugar into our mouths. Nor are we likely to dip our finger into lard or soft margarine and eat it straight. Straight alcohol is rarely consumed alone. Drinks are mixed, or alcohol is consumed as wine or beer, both of which have partial wholeness values. About the only group of nonwhole foods that we commonly do eat directly are processed grains, such as white flour in the form of white bread. Even then, we typically add fat (butter or margarine) and or sugar (jelly or straight sugar as in doughnuts or cookies).

With this exception of processed grains, the direct consumption of nonwhole foods is not the issue. *The partial replacement of whole food calories with nonwhole food calories to reduce cost, increase shelf life, and alter taste is where the nutrition chaos begins.* Recall the strawberry jam example: a cup of table sugar is added to a cup of strawberries and heated. This may sound innocent enough. Sadly, less than 10 percent of the nutritional wholeness remains. The nonwhole sugar has *diluted* the whole-food goodness of the high-water content fruit. A cup of sugar has 778 calories, while a cup of strawberries has only 48 calories. This means that 95 percent of the calories in strawberry jam come from sugar, and only 5 percent from whole strawberries! Dilution makes for deluded consumers!

How to Eat More Whole Foods

I am hoping by this point you want to eat more whole foods! Knowledge is the most powerful and sustainable motivator. Knowing that choosing whole foods increases your nutrient intake, lowers your glycemic load, helps you maintain a healthy weight, and reduces your predisposition to inflammation should jump-start your efforts.

If this is new territory for you, start gradually but work progressively. Replace sweetened foods with fruits and berries. Replace sodas and other soft drinks with 100 percent juices or filtered water (tastes better). Replace added fats with nuts and nut butters. Feel good about using nuts, peanuts, eggs, avoca-

dos, olives, cocoa, and any other wrongly scorned whole food. Replace white flour and rice with whole grains. Remove visible fat from grain-fed meats.

By choosing whole foods, you are simulating our ancestral diet. Our ancestors ate only whole foods. They had no choice. You do. In our modern food environment, you need an understanding of whole foods in order to direct your choices wisely. It is not difficult. It is an interesting challenge, in fact. The payoffs are many.

The biggest payoff is for those of you who are interested in controlling bad inflammation. Focusing on whole foods is the first and biggest step you can take toward balancing the inflammation that plagues you.

CHAPTER 9

BALANCING INFLAMMATION

If you are like me, there is a good chance you have turned to this chapter first. You are looking for answers. You are inflamed. It will not resolve. You want to know why.

Perhaps you are in pain. Arthritis pain. Fibromyalgia muscle pain. Chronic headache pain. Unrelenting back pain. The list of chronic pain syndromes is extensive.

Pain and inflammation go hand in hand. Pain is intended to be protective. It signals that an injured or infected part of the body needs attention and nurturing. Pain is that part's cry for help. It is a plea for special care in order to prevent further injury or the spread of infection. Pain should be part of a healing process.

When chronic inflammation sets in, the protective intent of pain loses its meaning. Chronic pain in the early stages is annoying. Without relief, the pain can shift to a kind of personal torment. Unrelenting pain is further amplified by despair and depression.

How is the downward spiral of chronic pain broken? As in all disease and illness, it is best to look for the underlying cause—find and correct it! Pain is one of the classic signs of inflammation. Inflammation causes pain. Bad inflammation causes chronic, unresolved pain.

Inflammation in and of itself is not "bad." Without inflammation our species could not have survived in the past, nor can we do so today. Inflammation is part of the body's natural ability to heal injury and prevent the spread of infection. Bad inflammation is a malfunction of this fundamental intent to heal. In essence, the process of healing has become sick. What can be done to restore balance to the inflammatory process? How is bad inflammation made good once again?

Five Pathways to Healing

My personal recovery from inflammatory rhinitis involved five pathways to healing that were woven into the early chapters of this guide. Paula and Gene's case studies contain elements of these five pathways, although no two people will have an identical story to tell. Healing is a very personal and individualized process.

The five pathways to healing are general dietary guidelines and lifestyle principles that find their true power when they are used together in a synergistic fashion. Each individual must discover her or his own unique blend of dietary change, adverse-food avoidance requirements, dietary supplements, and most important, each must have a "can-do" attitudinal shift. In other words, healing bad inflammation cannot be reduced to a simple recipe that fits all, or a single drug treatment. Lifestyle change is complex and varies tremendously—each patient is unique. The five pathways will help you get started. Enlisting the help of a nutritionally oriented health practitioner is another important step in this process.

The First Pathway: Whole Foods

Our ancestral diet was, by necessity, made up of foods available in the environment and therefore composed of 100 percent whole foods. This is the dietary environment in which our genes evolved. In a real sense, our genes are programmed to utilize whole foods. Several thousand years ago, the human species began deviating from this dietary blueprint. As carefully outlined in Chapter 5, Pro-inflammatory Dietary Shifts, the changes that have occurred in the way we eat have predisposed us to "bad" inflammation. The most fundamental "bad" change was the development of nonwhole foods: refined sugars, processed grains, and separated fats.

Nonwhole foods are invisible to most people. The shift to nonwhole foods has occurred slowly over the last 2,000 years of human culture. Nonwhole foods have been unconsciously assimilated into our very comprehension of what food is. So much so that most of us are totally unaware of their presence.

Strawberry jam now seems like a good way to eat strawberries. Ninety-five percent of the jam is sugar (0 percent whole), Doughnuts "naturally" go with coffee. Doughnuts are composed of white flour (50 percent whole), sugar (0 percent whole), and vegetable shortening (0 percent whole) with the added threat of trans fats, which are considered toxic antinutrients.

The idea of "diet" did not even exist in the minds of our ancestors. Food simply meant survival. Cells live a similar existence. Either they get the nutrients they need, or they do not. Either the full array of building-block nutrients are available or the cells begin to suffer degrees of starvation.

For our ancestors, starvation was a much quicker, more clear-cut phenomenon. A few weeks or months without adequate food, and they simply starved. In modern times, we get plenty of calories in the form of nonwhole foods. So we starve in a much different way from our ancestors. We suffer cellular nutrient starvation. Our cells do not calorie-starve. Our cells nutrient-starve. The process takes a lot longer—decades longer. Nutrient starvation takes the form of immune dysfunction, "bad" inflammation, connective tissue breakdown, insulin resistance and diabetes, heart disease, Alzheimer's disease, osteoporosis, tooth decay, and a whole host of diseases tied with degeneration and accelerated aging.

"Bad" inflammation appears to be a nutrient starvation phenomenon that gives rise to an imbalancing of the delicate sentinel function of inflammation. Choosing 80 to 90 percent of your foods as whole foods begins to reverse this cellular nutrient starvation. A whole foods diet consists of much more than meeting the RDAs. These numbers are minimum amounts. RDAs do not take into account the effects of decades of nonwhole foods diluting the nutrient content of the food you consume. *Orthomolecular vitamin and mineral supple-mentation* may be required to make up for lost time and lost nutrients. You can be tested for any hidden deficiencies.

Nonwhole foods are not "bad." People who eat non-whole foods (including you) are not "bad." "Bad" is a moral-istic judgment. Sugar is not a

> **Orthomolecular**
> *Literally means "right molecules." Using mole-cules that naturally occur in the body in larger than RDA doses to overcome genetic deficiencies.*

moral issue. It's a cellular-function issue. By compari-son, if you run out of gas, it doesn't make you "bad." It makes you walk.

Cells running low on key nutrients over long spans of time are not "bad" either. Such deficiencies make you feel tired. They set you up for infection. They make your cell membranes less responsive to insulin. They increase your risk of arteries plaquing up and blocking blood flow to vital organs. They predispose you to an excessive inflammatory response to injury or infection. These consequences are undesirable.

You can do better! Our ancestral diet is the key!

The Second Pathway: Lowering Your AA/EPA Ratio

Our ancestors ate a diet high in omega-3 fats. These fats are rich in eicosapentaenoic acid (EPA). EPA modulates and slows arachidonic acid's (AA's) con-version to pro-inflammatory eicosanoids. Animals that were hunted by our preagricultural ancestors ate a wide diversity of wild plants and animals, whose cells contained a rich reserve of omega-3 fats. The diverse supply of plant-related foods gathered by our ancestors was also a great source for omega-3 fats that favorably balanced their omega-6 fat con-tent. Fish and shellfish were especially good sources of omega-3.

That all changed with agriculture, when grains became the staple food. While still whole at this time in history, grains were abundant in omega-6 fats, thus beginning to tip the AA/EPA scale in the pro-inflammatory direction. It became easier to feed farm animals grains. Now their cellular omega-6 levels also went up at the expense of omega-3 levels. Milling and refining grains destroyed what little omega-3 grains contained. Finally, in more recent times, man-made trans fats were developed. Fast foods are cooked in trans fats. Trans fats actually act as an "anti-omega-3" factor that disrupts membrane function, including anti-inflammatory eicosanoid production.

By switching almost exclusively to whole foods, limiting wheat and other grains (especially if you have reason to think you could be allergic to them), and emphasizing range-fed meats and ocean fish, you can begin to reconstruct a much lower omega-6/omega-3 ratio in your cells. By adding orthomolecular doses of pharmaceutical-grade fish oil, you can greatly accelerate this process.

Obtain a fatty acid panel from a nutritionally oriented lab. Is your AA/EPA ratio about 20/1? If so, you have a pro-inflammatory disposition. Change your diet as prescribed above. Take pharmaceutical-grade fish oil as a supplement for a couple months. Start with one or two capsules per day. If you are not on Coumadin or heparin, work your way up to two per meal. One to two teaspoons of the straight oil is less expensive and can be taken once a day. If it is pharmaceutical grade, and you keep it refrigerated, the taste is a nonissue. You can also add it to a berry smoothie if desired.

Retest your AA/EPA ratio. Are you now approaching the ideal 3:1 ratio or lower? If yes, and if you are adopting the other pathways to healing, you should be noticing reductions in your "-itis" illnesses and symptoms. Overall, you will notice the emergence of a greater sense of well-being.

The Third Pathway: Lowering Your Glycemic Load

There are good carbs and there are bad carbs. Bad carbs tend to be white, starchy, sweet, low in fiber, quickly consumed, and highly processed, and they tend to enter your bloodstream very rapidly, usually as pure sugar molecules that stress your pancreas's ability to make insulin. Bad carbs form the backbone of America's convenience food industry. They have a very long shelf life. They appeal to taste. They can be eaten on the run. They have a very high glycemic index and trigger a big-time insulin response.

Here's the pattern: You like sweets. You wake up tired and unrefreshed from sleep. So you go for your usual cup of coffee, with sugar, and a doughnut for breakfast. That gets you going with the double whammy of caffeine and sugar. Your blood sugar sky-rockets. You head off to work while your pancreas struggles to produce the unnaturally large amount of insulin that is necessary to drive all that sugar into your cells. Well, it gets the job done—but overshoots in the amount of insulin it produces. Around 10:00 that morning, you feel shaky, irritable, headachy, and unable to concentrate. You make a beeline for the pop machine. A can of soda pop contains about nine teaspoons of sugar, plus more caffeine. You recover from the hypoglycemic reaction, long enough to get your morning's work done.

Again, your pancreas has "overreacted" and your blood sugar is roller coasting down a harrowing slope. Thank goodness it is time for lunch. Another coke, burger on a white bun, with a chocolate shake to go. Your blood sugar is once again catapulted into the stratosphere. What goes up must come down. This is why people complain of feeling sleepy after lunch. You go for an early coffee break, this time with an extra teaspoon of sugar. A few stale cookies left in the break room are snarfed down. The last few hours before heading home turn out to be wasted time: You just do not feel like accomplishing anything. Maybe beer and crackers at the bar will help.

This illustration may seem overly dramatic. But for millions of tired Americans, it is not. Hypoglycemia is only the beginning of a devastating decline in your cells ability to handle glucose. This decline in cellular membrane function can be diagnosed with a fasting insulin level. If it is high, you are headed for diabetes and increasing levels of inflammation.

High insulin levels favor the production of AA. This leads to a rise in the AA:EPA ratio in your cell membranes. Membrane function deteriorates. Insulin receptors malfunction. Your cells become resistant to insulin. The pancreas produces an even higher level of insulin. You begin to urinate copiously. You lose weight unexpectedly after years of gaining weight.

Your doctor diagnoses type 2 diabetes. You go on medication but fail to change your diet. Eventually your pancreas "burns out." You are required to go on insulin. You notice numbness in your feet (diabetic neuropathy). Your vision deteriorates (diabetic retinopathy). You have a heart attack (increased risk for plaque formation). Your kidneys fail (diabetic nephropathy). Amputations are required (diabetes plugs blood vessels and blocks blood flow to feet and hands). The eventual death of a diabetic can be quite gruesome.

If you are showing signs of hypoglycemia or Syndrome X (like Paula in Chapter 6), wake up now! You can change this pattern for the better! Start paying attention to glycemic index and glycemic load. These numbers are available free on the Internet. Simply type in the web address for a search engine such as Google (www.google.com), and type in *glycemic index* or *glycemic load* to find several useful sites that offer complete listings of these values for common foods.

Remember that the deeper and richer the natural color of the food item, the lower is its glycemic impact. Some have referred to this as *the color code*. This is a whole foods shortcut that can help you make better food choices when you don't have time to look up the numbers.

The Fourth Pathway: Raising Your ORAC Score

The color code also points to the high ORAC foods. As you may recall, ORAC stands for Oxidant Radical Absorbance Capacity. It is a standardized measurement of a food's ability to absorb and neutralize damaging free radicals. Whole, colorful foods are rich in natural antioxidants. Antioxidants protect your cells and their components from the corrosive effect of oxygen free radicals. These are what make metal rust, cut apples turn brown, cataracts form in your eye's lens, and brown lipofuscin (liver) spots form on your skin, to name just a few examples.

One effect of bad inflammation is the excessive cytokine stimulation of white blood cells to form lysozymes. These enzymes were meant to clean up the cellular debris resulting from injury or infection. Lysozymes release peroxide to clean up wounds in much the same way you and I would pour hydrogen peroxide in a cut or abrasion to disinfect it. Just the right amount works great. Too much and the excessive free radicals end up damaging vital tissues.

You can also take antioxidant supplements. Vitamins C and E are famous for their water- and fat-soluble antioxidant power. Coenzyme Q_{10}, alpha lipoic acid, n-acetyl cysteine, and a host of lesser-known nutrients can also supplement your whole food sources. Herbal compounds, long respected for their healing powers, are actually concentrated phytonutrients with powerful antioxidant effects. Tea contains catechins; tomatoes boast lycopene; and grape seed extract is rich in proanthocyanidins. There are many wonderful whole plant extracts that can be used to boost your daily ORAC consumption and lower the damage from excessive cytokine activity. Herbal seasonings are rich ORAC sources also.

The Fifth Pathway: Eliminating Reactive Foods

The phrase *food allergy means* different things to different medical specialists. An allergist considers only severe allergic reactions, such as anaphylactic shock or severe hives from eating peanuts or strawberries, as a true food allergy. Yet most people know that certain foods cause certain negative reactions in their bodies that an allergist would not call *food allergies.*

I'm referring to a spectrum of highly individual reactions that people can have to food. This means that not everyone responds the same way. For example, a more innocuous food reaction is sneezing with a drink of wine. This is not a typical food allergy; it is an *adverse food reaction* (AFR)—and a mild one at that. What about getting a migraine after you eat blue cheese? Again, that is an adverse food reaction. MSG (monosodium glutamate) can also trigger headaches, but not in everyone. Many foods can trigger headaches, but whether they do or not depends on the individual response, and that can be highly unpredictable.

Many more examples can be given of unique individual responses, in uniquely adverse ways, to a variety of food triggers. How is this phenomenon explained, and what does it have to do with healing bad inflammation?

The genesis of adverse food reactions can be found within the origins of bad inflammation itself. The pro-inflammatory dietary shifts that have occurred over the last several millennia have resulted in the development of chronic inflammation in the gut. Nonwhole foods have weakened the cellular function of *enterocytes* (the cells that line the gut). The gut is lined with a trillion live bacteria that form the friendly flora of the gut. These and an estimated 80 percent of the body's entire population of white blood cells patrol the surface area of the gut, which is equal to that of two tennis courts! Viruses, bacteria, parasites, fungi, toxins, and a host of potential threats enter the arena of the gut with each and every feeding. All of these can act as triggers to the inflammatory process. With a progressive loss of whole-food nutrients, a rise in pro-inflammatory omega-6 at the expense of anti-inflammatory omega-3, a barrage of glycemic-dysregulating refined sugars and starches, and a paucity of antioxidant ORAC foods, the lining of the gut becomes a prime target for the progressive development of bad inflammation.

Remember that the third microscopic step of acute inflammation is *mobilize*! The release of cytokines loosens the junctions between endothelial cells, including enterocytes. Peptides leak into the bloodstream before they are broken down to amino acids.

Too big to cross cell membranes, these protein fragments roam the bloodstream until lymphocytes start making antibodies against them. Antibodies clump to peptides and form immune complexes. These complexes will accumulate in the basement membranes of various organs, depending upon unique individual factors such as prior injury or infection, genetic predisposition, even psychological factors ("I can't stomach this marriage," "This job is one big headache").

Adverse food reactions are a common cause of low-grade, systemic inflammation. By identifying your AFRs through blood testing or elimination diets you can *unload* a major contributor to bad inflammation in your body.

A couple simple techniques to try out in your search to identify AFRs:

1. Take out a piece of paper and write down your ten most favorite foods or beverages. These are the ones you crave and eat frequently. Chances are that at least five of the ten will be significant AFRs. Try eliminating one or more of these foods for a couple weeks and see how you feel.

2. Try eating *monomeals*. These are meals composed of only one food. Then do the pulse test. Count your pulse before eating. (Count your wrist or neck pulse for fifteen seconds and multiply times four.) Then ten to fifteen minutes after your monomeal, count your pulse again. If your pulse increases by more than five to ten beats per minute, you may be having an AFR.

Blocking versus Healing

Relief from symptoms usually drives those of us in pain to medication. Anti-inflammatory meds do relieve pain. The anti-inflammatory meds do not, however, distinguish between bad and good inflammation. The long-term side effects from NSAIDs are well documented. These highly touted COX enzyme inhibitors can cause stomach pain, ulcers, and bleeding. Other more serious side effects, including heart attack, kidney damage, and heart failure, have also been linked to these meds. A startling statistic: One-fifth of the 5 million American cases of heart failure may be related to NSAID usage.

Medication works by blocking key biochemical pathways in the body. They work fast and often provide symptom relief. The long-term price to be paid comes in side effects and toxic drug interactions.

Nutrients feed biochemical pathways, healing and enhancing cellular function. Symptoms resolve slowly but progressively, based upon a true correction of the underlying issues. Often there are side benefits. Using nutrients as therapy frees you from the worry of long-term toxic reactions.

Recall my futile attempts to suppress the symptoms of my own case of inflammatory rhinitis. They helped but did not heal. Using the five pathways of healing gave me long-term resolution of my illness, and better overall health.

CHAPTER 10

INFLAMAGING

An important risk factor for heart disease is age. The older you are the more likely you are to get a heart attack. The same is true for stroke and cancer. Arthritis increases with age. In general, chronic degenerative illness is more likely to occur the older you are.

This is not a new revelation. Our life experience tells us that getting old is often associated with disease and disability. Aging and disease go hand in hand.

What may be new is the emerging scientific realization that "bad" inflammation is a major *common denominator*. Inflammation is no longer seen as a localized, organ-specific phenomenon. Low-grade, systemic inflammation has been identified as a fundamental mechanism driving both chronic degenerative disease and aging.

New Evidence for InflamAging

Dr. C. Franceschi and colleagues from Italy have coined the term *inflamm-Aging* to highlight this important connection between "bad" inflammation and age-associated degenerative disease. The elderly have increased levels of pro-inflammatory cytokines. IL-6, IL-1, tumor necrosis factor, and interferon gamma are examples of pro-inflammatory cytokines that increase with age. Anti-inflammatory cytokines, like interferon alpha and beta, decrease with age.

IL-6 is a pro-inflammatory cytokine that plays a role in heart disease, osteoporosis, and Alzheimer's disease. It is barely detectable in young, healthy people. With the aging process, IL-6 levels increase significantly. Elderly female heart patients with the highest levels of IL-6 were four times more likely to die in the next three years compared to those with the lowest levels of IL-6. Higher levels of IL-6 put the elderly at higher risk for cognitive decline, loss of muscle mass and strength, and earlier onset of disability.

Aging is the sum total of a lifetime of injuries, infections, acquired allergies, and free-radical damage—all of which serve as chronic inflammatory triggers. Nutrient deficiencies, nonwhole food consumption, low omega-3 intake, high glycemic load, and the intake of low ORAC-score foods further predispose us to low-level inflammation, both chronic and systemic.

Ironically, while "stealth inflammation" builds with aging, inflammatory responsiveness gradually becomes more blunted. The elderly are more prone to serious infections, like flu and pneumonia. This blunted responsiveness may be self-protective. InflamAging may involve the biological attempt to counterbalance the buildup of pro-inflammatory cytokines with down-regulated inflammatory responsiveness. If the elderly can avoid overwhelming stress, such as an operation, injury, or major infection, they can live fairly well in spite of rising levels of pro-inflammatory cytokines.

Beyond Pharmacology

It is all too common to visit an ailing elder in a nursing home or care facility only to discover they are taking ten or more medications. Because of declining liver and renal clearance, the elderly are at higher risk for drug toxicity. Add to this the heightened risk of drug interactions. Yet it is the frail elderly who most commonly experience polypharmacy, as doctors heroically attempt to control their mounting symptoms and suffering.

Polypharmacy
The administration of an excessive number of drugs with a higher likelihood of interactions and side effects.

The understanding that "bad" inflammation is at the root of "diseases of the aged" identifies an alternative to polypharmacy. The five pathways to healing chronic inflammation address the biological origins of the problem. Using drugs to treat a diet-related disorder will offer temporary relief at best, and side effects at worst. The recent recall of Vioxx illustrates this.

The *User's Guide to Inflammation, Arthritis, and Aging* offers a *bio-logical* answer to inflamAging that could be applied to old and young alike. Dr. Boyd Eaton's discovery that our ancestors were free of degenerative disease is cause for hope. The five pathways to healing recreate our ancestral diet and its inflammation-balancing capabilities. The pathways combine rational dietary modification with special supplementation to recreate and amplify the advantages of our ancestral diet. The five pathways are an effective means of controlling inflammation without the risky side effects of NSAIDs and other symptom-reducing medications.

By introducing the five pathways at a young age and pursuing them diligently throughout life, one can reduce their cumulative "inflammatory load" and literally slow the inflamAging process! This could effectively reduce our societal dread of aging. Low inflammatory elders could live and function as youngsters if their inflammatory systems were properly balanced throughout the span of their lifetimes. Hundreds of dreaded "-itis" diseases would be avoided. Medication and hospitalization costs would be reduced. An era of balanced inflammation would see a society relatively free of chronic illness, where the high cost of sickness care would be funneled into optimal health research, optimal nutrition programs, optimal fitness standards, environmental toxicity reduction, and a focus on creating what really matters to each of us as unique individuals.

Is this a utopian vision? Yes, but only if you wait for conventional thinkers to bless it. Why not give it a try yourself right now? It can't hurt. Become a colearner now. Take charge of your life, your health, and your inflammatory system. The key to balance lies within you. Use it to open the door to a better life!

CONCLUSION

Inflammation is the body's protective, healing response to injury and infection. As a sentinel, it is on alert and ready to be activated when triggered. Anti-inflammatory regulators balance these powerful pro-inflammatory forces. This dynamic equilibrium has served us well over the course of our species' evolution. In this sense, inflammation is "good."

With the advent of agriculture, major shifts away from the diet of our ancestors were underway, and these shifts disrupted the balance of forces. High omega-6 grains and the loss of a diverse array of protective ORAC foods began to favor a pro-inflammatory predisposition in the body. The industrial revolution gave mankind the ability to process foods on a large scale. Sugar factories, grain mills, and huge oil presses made cheap nonwhole foods widely available. The modern rush to convenience foods enculturated a food supply with less than half the nutritional value of our original diet—the rest had been stripped away. Food sensitivities became commonplace, glycemic loads soared, and the antioxidant capabilities of foods plummeted. The high omega-6/omega-3 ratio of these foods favored the emergence of epidemics of "bad" inflammation illness.

The recent withdrawal of a major anti-inflammatory pharmaceutical agent from the marketplace due to unacceptable side effects marks a shift in our national consciousness. There is no quick-fix way to solve a problem that has its origins in the way we eat. If "bad" inflammation is primarily a dietary problem, as this health guide suggests it is, then the "problem" will be solved by a societal rediscovery of its ancestral diet—a diet based in whole foods, rich in omega-3 fats and high ORAC plant edibles, and low in the dismembered, dysglycemic grains and sugars that dysregulate our blood glucose levels, inflame our gastrointestinal tracts, and promote the development of adverse food reactions.

InflamAging finds its origins in the wide societal disregard for our ancestral diet. Chronic inflammation slowly progresses to low-grade, systemic inflammation. Clusters of degenerative diseases emerge. Aging is accelerated. Medical costs skyrocket. Premature aging and death become the norm.

By adopting the five pathways to healing, we are able to recreate our ancestral diet in modern times. Anti-inflammatory regulators once again balance the pro-inflammatory forces. Systemic inflammation lessens. Chronic inflammation finally heals. Health is restored.

This *User's Guide to Inflammation, Arthritis, and Aging* is your guide to restoring inflammatory health. To heal any health problem, the acutal underlying causes must be addressed and corrected. When these improvements are made permanent in your lifestyle, you can begin to live to your full genetic potential.

I wish you well!

SELECTED
REFERENCES

Berk B.C., Liuzzo G., and Ridker PM. C-reactive protein: A "golden marker" for inflammation and coronary artery disease. *Cleveland Clinic Journal of Medicine*, 2001;68(6): 521–534.

Davis, Donald R. Omega-3 fatty acids in clinical practice. *Journal of Advancement in Medicine*, 1995; 8(1):5–35.

Eaton, S. Boyd, and Konner, Melvin. Paleolithic nutrition. *The New England Journal of Medicine*, 1985; 312(5):283–289.

Franceschi C., Bonafe M., Valensin S., et al. Inflamm-aging. An evolutionary perspective on immunosenescence. *Annals of the New York Academy of Sciences*, 2000; 908:244–254.

Liuzzo, Giovanna, Biasucci, Luigi M., Gallimore, J. Ruth, et al. The prognostic value of c-reactive protein and serum amyloid a protein in severe unstable angina. *The New England Journal of Medicine*, 1994; 331(7):417–424.

Lopez-Garcia, Esther, Schulze, Matthias, Fung, Teresa T., et al. Major dietary patterns are related to plasma concentrations of markers of inflammation and endothelial dysfunction. *American Journal of Clinical Nutrition*, 2004; 80:1029–1035.

Muhlestein, Joseph B., Anderson, Jeffrey L., Hammond, Elizabeth H., et al. Infection with *Chlamydia pneumoniae* accelerates the development of atherosclerosis and treatment with azithromycin prevents it in a rabbit model. *Circulation*, 1998; 97:633–636.

Ridker P. M., Hennekens C. H., Buring J. E., et al.. C-reactive protein and other markers of inflammation in the prediction of cardiovascular disease in women. *The New England Journal of Medicine*, 2000; 342(12):836–843.

Rooney, P.J. et al. A short review of the relationship between intestinal permeability and inflammatory joint disease. *Clinical and Experimental Rheumatology*, 1990; 8:75–83.

Yeh, Edward T.H., and Willerson, James T. Coming of age of c-reactive protein. *Circulation*, 2003; 107:370–372.

OTHER BOOKS AND RESOURCES

Challem, Jack. *The Inflammation Syndrome*. Hoboken, NJ: Wiley, 2003.

Challem, Jack, Berkson, Burton and Smith, Melissa Diane. *Syndrome X*. New York: Wiley, 2000.

Deron, Scott J. *C-reactive Protein*. New York: Contemporary Books, 2004.

Lipski, Elizabeth. *Leaky Gut Syndrome*. Los Angeles: Keats, 1998.

Macleod, A.G. *Aspects of Acute Inflammation*. Kalamazoo, MI: Upjohn, 1973.

Meggs, William Joel, and Svec, Carol. *The Inflammation Cure*. New York: Contemporary Books, 2004.

Reaven, Gerald, Strom, Terry Kirsten, and Fox, Barry. *Syndrome X: The Silent Killer*. New York: Fireside, 2000.

Sears, Barry. *The Omega Rx Zone*. New York: HarperCollins, 2002.

GreatLife Magazine
Consumer magazine with articles on vitamins, minerals, herbs, and foods.

Available for free at many health and natural food stores.

Let's Live Magazine
Consumer magazine with emphasis on the health benefits of vitamins, minerals, and herbs.

Customer service:
1-800-676-4333
P.O. Box 74908
Los Angeles, CA 90004

Subscriptions: 12 issues per year, $19.95 in the U.S.; $31.95 outside the U.S.

Physical Magazine

Magazine oriented to body builders and other serious athletes.

Customer service:

1-800-676-4333

P.O. Box 74908

Los Angeles, CA 90004

Subscriptions: 12 issues per year, $19.95 in the U.S.;
$31.95 outside the U.S.

The Nutrition Reporter™ newsletter

Monthly newsletter that summarizes recent medical research on vitamins, minerals, and herbs.

Customer service:

P.O. Box 30246

Tucson, AZ 85751-0246

e-mail: jack@thenutritionreporter.com

www.nutritionreporter.com

Subscriptions: $26 per year (12 issues) in the U.S.;
$32 U.S. or $48 CNC for Canada; $38 for other countries

The Center for the Improvement of Human Functioning International

www.brightspot.org

The Inflammation Syndrome

www.inflammationsyndrome.com

Feed Your Genes Right

www.feedyourgenesright.com

INDEX